INTERNAL AUDITING FOR HOSPITALS

Seth Allcorn

Aspen Systems Corporation
Germantown, Maryland
London, England
1979

Library of Congress Cataloging in Publication Data

Allcorn, Seth.
Internal auditing for hospitals.

Includes bibliographical references and index.
1. Hospitals—Accounting. 2. Hospitals—Auditing and
inspection. 3. Auditing, Internal.
I. Title.
HF5686.H7A44 657'.832 79-20072
ISBN 0-89443-163-3

Library of Congress Catalog Card Number: 79-20072
ISBN: 0-89443-163-3

Printed in the United States of America

1 2 3 4 5

Table of Contents

Preface

This book is written with the firm belief that modern internal auditing must be adopted by the health care industry. The nature of the industry, hospitals, and physicians is such that good administration and cost control has become difficult, and promises to become more so as new demands are made by government and the public for more economical management of the nation's health care resources. The purpose of this book is to advocate internal auditing in all hospitals, regardless of size.

The practice of modern internal auditing holds many benefits for hospitals and the public. Internal auditing will help hospitals improve efficiency and effectiveness, will spot wastes and poor administrative practices, and will recommend changes in operating procedures to enhance internal control of all business and patient care activities. Hospitals can recover the cost of their investment in the function many times over as their operations become progressively better controlled because of the single-minded efforts of internal auditors. Hospitals not contemplating the addition of an internal auditor must not be without the capability. The basic precepts of internal auditing must be practiced by hospital administrators.

With this in mind, the book includes the perspective of hospital directors to encourage themselves to conduct internal auditing and, in doing so, to recognize eventually the necessity for formally staffing the function. The word function, rather than internal auditing department, is used throughout to recognize its embryonic state in the health care industry. Hospitals that have had internal auditing for years may have had time to evolve a distinct department with a staff and a director. For the rest of the industry, the goal of a completely staffed department of internal auditing is premature and must wait until perhaps the 21st century. Nonetheless, hospitals must begin now to develop internal auditing vigorously to meet even this goal.

The book is arranged to provide basic readings in theory and practice and detailed discussions of practical applications. In this regard, this is a synthesis of a wide assortment of published material on hospital administration, hospital financial management, hospital internal auditing, and internal auditing and management in general. Much care is given to avoid implicit inclusions of schools of thought that the reader, being unaware of, would not recognize. Every effort is made to present generally accepted principles for internal auditing. Where necessary, additional points of view are inserted to promote critical thinking. A key component of the chapters dealing with practical applications is that none of the discussions and audit checklists is exhaustive. Administrators and internal auditors will recognize readily that a checklist for any activity always is incomplete and not all points are applicable to all situations. There generally is substantial literature on subjects under study and auditors should read this material as background in preparation for designing their investigative programs. These factors apply to all the lists of checkpoints throughout this volume and, in the interest of avoiding needless repetition, are not restated before each list. Readers are encouraged, when using this text in practical situations, to examine other sections and chapters for potentially related points and not to stop there but to continue to think critically and add to the list from their own observations.

It is my hope, as the author, that this work contributes to expanding the service role internal auditing can play in hospitals and, by doing so, permits the function to contribute to improving the health care delivery system.

Acknowledgments

It is a pleasure to recognize the efforts of those who have helped and inspired me in the preparation of this book. I am especially grateful to Charles E. Mengel, M.D., Chairman of the Department of Medicine of the University of Missouri-Columbia, for providing me the incentive and opportunity to pursue my interest in hospital internal auditing and hospital management.

I am grateful to Robert Boissoneau, Dean of the College of Human Services, Eastern Michigan University; William Sedgeman, Sr., Director of Internal Auditing at Owens-Corning Fiberglass (Retired) and currently a consultant to hospitals implementing internal auditing departments; and Harold Boyer, Director of Internal Auditing and Records Management for the University of Missouri-Columbia who provided many helpful comments and criticisms during the writing of the book.

I owe a debt to Sally Coats who competently typed the rough drafts and final copy of the manuscript and other members of the Department of Medicine who contributed to the writing and revising of the manuscript.

Last, I am grateful to my wife Mary for her expert assistance in preparing the index and for generally tolerating my absences during the writing of the book.

Part I

Foundations of Internal Auditing in Hospitals

Chapter 1

Modern Internal Auditing

The health care industry must provide good service at a reasonable cost. Boards of directors, physicians, and hospital administrators must begin diligently to seek improved health care while trying to contain rising costs. Thus far in the pursuit of this goal, an entire field of endeavor is untapped by hospitals—that of modern internal auditing. Modern internal auditing is a proved function on which most industries have come to rely. The absence of internal auditing in most of the 7,000 hospitals in the United States is a fact that must be recognized by today's generation of board members and administrators.

For the health care industry to develop internal auditing to an extent that it can realize operating benefits, board members, hospital administrators, and auditors must understand what the function is and what services it can contribute to an institution's operations. The first four chapters provide a condensed discussion of the art of internal auditing. Board members and administrators should read on through Chapter 9 to learn specifics of internal auditing. They must learn that internal auditing is not something new; it is a fully developed profession. They must know that most major industries have employed internal auditing successfully for decades. Finally, they must be aware that a well-conceived and fully utilized program of internal auditing can earn its way by contributing to the improvement of management controls and operations over the broad spectrum of functions and activities that comprise today's modern hospital.[1]

A word on terminology and how top management and middle management are used: Top management includes the hospital director or president and all assistant administrators who participate in the overall management of the institution. Depending on the context, top management also may include the governing board. Hospital administration refers to the director and assistant administrators. Middle management includes department managers and their administrative assistants. Hospital director is used instead of president. Department refers to discrete hospital activities usually given departmental status. Function means activities not usually provided department status or performed in common by many departments.

INTERNAL AUDITING'S NATURE

Many scholars have dealt with the nature of internal auditing, however, none improve upon The Institute of Internal Auditors' new *Standards for the Professional Practice of Internal Auditing*:

> Internal auditing is an independent appraisal function established within an organization to examine and evaluate its activities as a service to the organization. The objective of internal auditing is to assist members of the organization in the effective discharge of their responsibilities. To this end, internal auditing furnishes them with analyses, appraisals, recommendations, counsel, and information concerning the activities reviewed[2] (Appendix A).

The Institute of Internal Auditors is the principle professional organization within the field of internal auditing and is the only organization with a certification program for internal auditors. The above statement presents clearly and concisely the Institute's conception of the nature of internal auditing. Internal auditing:

- Is an independent appraisal function. Independence is essential for the effective functioning of internal auditing. Internal auditing must be free of organizational constraints and pressures and must not compromise its objectivity by participating directly in management. The internal auditing function fulfills its role by appraising the activities performed by the hospital in relation to stated goals and objectives and by making recommendations and pertinent comments about the usefulness of the activities reviewed.
- Exists within an organization. Internal auditing does not resemble the auditing of certified public accountants, although both are auditors and both share many common methods and techniques. Public accountants are concerned primarily with validating the accuracy and representativeness of hospital financial statements, whereas internal auditing is management- and operations-oriented and, in that regard, is interested in assisting the hospital in achieving its goals.
- Examines and evaluates its activities as a service to the organization. The scope of a hospital's operational components that can be audited is limited only by top management restrictions, and by the auditor's imagination, inquiring mind, and ability. Internal auditors may find they are restricted to the traditional area of financial auditing, a protective appraisal of financial matters using commonly accepted concepts of control for comparison. No effort is made to evaluate the operation further in terms of its relation to other elements of the hospital and its overall contribution to the institution's

goals. An appraisal of this scope, which may include financial auditing, is an operations audit. Operations auditing is an evolving appraisal activity for which no practitioner as yet has put forward an accepted definition. (See Chapter 4 for attempted definitions.) Operations auditing assumes a top management perspective; that is, it specifically attempts to enhance all parts of the hospital that contribute to fulfilling its goals and seeks out, for evaluation, organizational elements that act as a drain on resources by not contributing to the goals. To accomplish this, the auditor will appraise the managerial organization, all levels of staffing and work performance, communication and information systems, and general management operating controls.[3] It should be understood clearly that although internal auditing reports to top management and the governing board and essentially assumes a top management orientation in its reviews, it must not be lost sight of that the goal of both top management and internal auditing is service to the hospital.[4]

- Assists members of the organization in the effective discharge of their responsibilities. Internal auditors are responsible to all levels of management for providing information about the adequacy and effectiveness of the hospital's system of internal control. Administrators and department managers are responsible for internal control in their areas and, in fact, depend on good internal control to manage today's larger and more complex hospitals. Internal control is the product of a sound managerial organization that provides for constant measuring and evaluation of: (1) the representativeness and accuracy of data and reports, (2) the overall efficiency of the organization, and (3) the degree to which organizational participants follow policies and procedures.[5] Internal auditing is one of the major ingredients of the total concept of internal control. Because of its independent organizational status, internal auditing is able to make objective evaluations of internal control and performance.

- Furnishes management with analyses, appraisals, recommendations, counsel, and information concerning the activities reviewed. Internal auditors report to all levels of management, including the department manager, the administrator responsible for the department, the hospital director, and the governing board or its audit committee. The internal auditor is responsible for documenting all findings adequately in a professional, objective manner. Recommendations must have been researched thoroughly and talked through with managers at the level of implementation. An important point that may be overlooked easily is that it is not sufficient merely to report accurate and useful findings and recommendations; the auditor is responsible for convincing top management of their worth. The auditor's work is complete only when recommendations are implemented. It is apparent that internal auditing can be described This is an important part of being recognized as a responsible and useful function and profession. The nature of internal auditing is universal and can benefit any type of organization that has defined goals. It must also be stated that internal auditing should not become another amoral bureaucratic instrument; rather, it must exert a positive moral influence on the hospital. Internal auditing is ideally suited for providing modern hospitals, large or small, a means of improving patient care, containing costs, and developing adequate and meaningful internal controls. Internal auditing can easily and effectively perform in an organization type—the hospital—that is regarded by students of organization as one of the most advanced organizational structures in existence today.[6]

HISTORICAL EVOLUTION OF INTERNAL AND OPERATIONS AUDITING

Internal auditing has an interesting history that helps provide perspective for understanding its nature.

The function—not the profession—of internal auditing existed during the earliest civilizations. There is historical evidence of the use of internal auditing techniques during early Mesopotamian civilization (3600 to 3200 B.C.). It is known that the treasury of the Egyptian Pharaohs used internal auditing and that the Greeks and Romans by 500 B.C. had made extensive use of the function as a control over such government activities as tax collection.[7]

Internal auditing diminished as Rome fell and the early Middle Ages reversed the path of commercial progress by reverting to barter systems (300 to 600 A.D.). As the early Middle Ages grew to a close, however, there were the rudimentary beginnings of more advanced forms of commerce and government.[8]

By 1300 A.D., private enterprise was making rapid strides toward more complicated business units. Partnerships were being formed, creating increased dependence on records and accountability. Double entry bookkeeping was evolving in Italy as a vastly improved form of a control over transactions. Although improved bookkeeping techniques assisted merchants greatly with control, internal auditing still played an active role. Audits were being performed more frequently and on larger economic units, such as cities. Formal concepts of internal control such as specific types of internal checks also were evolving.[9]

During the early 1600s, the remnants of feudalism were disappearing in Europe and small towns and factories were springing up. Profit and loss and accountability assumed a new meaning to the new and larger business enterprises. By the 19th century, the size and complexity of enterprises and the creation of publicly owned corporations acted together to establish firmly the need for internal auditing practices.[10]

By the 20th century, reliance on internal auditing appeared to be the natural result of perceived need for management control by heads of government or managers. Once the size and complexity of an organization grew beyond the ability of the owner or manager to oversee it personally, there originated a need for a better system of control and ultimately for a person responsible for ensuring that the controls were effective and working. The early focus of internal auditing was on gaining control of an organization's finances and on detecting and preventing fraud. This became the traditional role up to the 1940s.

The mid-1940s saw the recognition of operations auditing as a distinct appraisal activity of internal auditing. Provision for operations auditing was made in the Institute of Internal Auditors' *Statement of Responsibilities of the Internal Auditor*. Under the heading of "Nature" it states, "It deals primarily with accounting and financial matters but it may also properly deal with matters of an operating nature."[11] With this formal recognition of both financial and operational internal auditing, the present era of modern internal auditing was born.

INTERNAL AUDITING: A BUDDING PROFESSION

As a profession, internal auditing has come a long way and owes much of its development to the diligent efforts of the Institute of Internal Auditors, Inc., formed in 1941. Other outside organizations also have contributed to the growth and recognition of internal auditing as a profession. The Securities and Exchange Commission and the American Institute of Certified Public Accountants both have recognized its importance and have supported its growth actively.[12]

Is internal auditing a profession? Dictionary definitions usually state that a profession is a vocation or occupation requiring advanced training or education in a specialized field. Internal auditing does require advanced training and education. A profession also has demonstrable attributes, such as:

- Statements of standards (Appendix A) and responsibilities (Appendix B)
- A code of ethics (Appendix C)
- A common body of knowledge (Appendix D)
- Certification programs
- Provision for continuing education
- A professional organization with a governing board

The Institute of Internal Auditors has fulfilled all these criteria and continues to review and improve on past work.

But there is more to a profession than simply meeting accepted criteria. There is the need for acceptance by the users, by academia, and by the public.[13] There is the need for a professional identity. Questions that internal auditors must answer are:

- Does top management accept and value their counsel?
- Does top management act on their recommendations?
- Does top management provide them enough independence to be objective?

A "no" answer is a strong indicator that the top management of the hospital has not yet accepted internal auditing as a profession. Internal auditors must renew efforts to convince top management of the function's professionalism, demonstrating through performance that it does contribute to the achievement of the hospital's goals. They should ask:

- Do colleges and universities teach internal auditing?
- Do academicians know of internal auditing and accept it as a profession?

Thus far, internal auditing has not been recognized widely by institutions of higher education as course material nor are faculties well informed about the subject.[14] Improvement has been slow but steady, with the Institute of Internal Auditors again leading the way.[15] Improvement should continue more rapidly as the federal government and the public insist on improved internal controls in all health care organizations. A final question:

- Is the general public aware of internal auditing as a profession?

The answer is "no." Public awareness is important in terms of receiving full recognition; however, such awareness is acquired only slowly, if at all. The public usually learns of internal auditing through its absence. Major instances of loss of internal control such as fraud cases or vast wastes of resources attract publicity. The public may learn of internal auditing's professional role in control as a result of demanding that such losses be stopped.

A last aspect of professionalism is a commitment by all members to seek excellence in the function.[16] The internal auditing manager and individual auditor must manage the function, including all of its component parts, properly. Lapses in excellence anywhere throughout the process detract from the remaining parts that are performed with excellence. Excellence also will help convince both management and the academic community that internal auditing is a needed and legitimate profession.

CONCLUSION

Internal auditing is a universal function that represents hospital and top management interests within the institution's overall internal control environment. The function assumes a management perspective as it appraises the effectiveness of a hospital's internal controls and operations. The ultimate goal of internal auditing is to provide service to the hospital so it can accomplish its goals better.

Internal control and internal auditing have had a long history based on the evolving need by leaders of large organizations for better control. Within the complex organizational environment of modern hospitals, internal auditing is a function uniquely adapted to provide improvements in management control and general operations.

NOTES

1. M. Humphrey, "Why Your Hospital Needs Internal Auditing," *Hospital Financial Management*, June 1971, p. 15.

2. The Institute of Internal Auditors, *Standards for the Professional Practice of Internal Auditing* (Altamonte Springs, Florida: The Institute of Internal Auditors, Inc., May 1978).

3. Dale L. Flesher, *Operations Auditing in Hospitals* (Lexington, Mass.: Lexington Books, 1976), p. 2.

4. The Institute of Internal Auditors, "Exposure Draft of the Standards for the Professional Practice of Internal Auditing," *Internal Auditor*, December 1977, p. 13.

5. Victor Z. Brink and James A. Cashin, *Internal Auditing* (New York: The Ronald Press Company, 1958), p. 10.

6. Wolf Heydebrand, *Hospital Bureaucracy: A Comparative Study of Organizations* (New York: Dunellen Publishing Co., 1973), p. xxv.

7. T. A. Lee, "The Historical Development of Internal Control from the Earliest Times to the End of the Seventeenth Century," *Journal of Accounting Research*, Spring 1971, p. 151.

8. Ibid., p. 154.

9. Ibid., pp. 155–156.

10. A. H. Adelberg, "Auditing on the March: Ancient Times to the Twentieth Century," *Internal Auditor*, December 1975, p. 37.

11. The Institute of Internal Auditors, *Increasing the Usefulness of Internal Auditing* (New York: The Institute of Internal Auditors, Inc.), 1948, p. 4.

12. Victor Z. Brink, James A. Cashin, and Herbert Witt, *Modern Internal Auditing: An Operational Approach* (New York: The Ronald Press Company, 1973), p. 4.

13. J. G. Morton, "The Professional Internal Auditor: Fact or Fantasy?" *Internal Auditor*, December 1974, p. 4.

14. Ibid., p. 48.

15. S. C. Gross, "Extend Internal Audit Influence," *Internal Auditor*, October 1976, pp. 16–19.

16. L. B. Sawyer, "Professionalism in Internal Auditing," *Internal Auditor*, February 1976, p. 17.

Chapter 2

Standards of Independence, Scope, and Performance

Internal auditing in hospitals must be governed by established standards of practice to ensure the institution's board and administration that the work is well managed, accurate, comprehensive, complete, and objective. Members of the board, administrators, and internal auditors must agree on mutually acceptable standards of performance. The Institute of Internal Auditors has prepared comprehensive standards that hospitals should adopt (Appendix A). The standards are a guide for judging independence and establish criteria for determining internal auditing's scope and evaluating its performance.

INDEPENDENCE

Independence is an especially important topic. Internal auditors must have independence from most hospital departments and high-ranking staff members to fulfill their function. Every hospital that has or is planning to add internal auditing should examine thoroughly the provisions it has made for independence. A health care institution is ill-advised to invest heavily in any function and fail to provide the basic tools for performance. It also should be noted that certified public accounting firms will depend on a hospital's internal auditors in direct proportion to the extent the CPA personnel perceive that the in-house staff has independence. The more the CPA firm can rely on a hospital's internal auditors, the less its engagement will cost.[1]

Independence exists where the internal auditing function receives proper organizational status and the means to maintain objectivity. "The organizational status of the internal audit department should be sufficient to permit the accomplishment of its audit responsibilities."[2] Internal auditors must be supported by top management and board members in order to be free from influence and in-

11

terference from hospital departments and to receive the cooperation of the institution's staff.

The Institute of Internal Auditors has specified six standards of practice for organizational status. First, internal auditing must report to a position high enough in the hospital that virtually all the rest of the institution falls under the control of that position. This will promote independence, ensure that auditing is free to review all aspects of the hospital and provide for adequate consideration of findings and effective responses to recommendations. In small and medium-sized institutions, internal auditing should report to the hospital's director and perhaps to the board if it meets frequently enough and has the time and the interest to examine actual operations. For larger institutions, internal auditing should report to the hospital's director, with direct communication privileges to the board or to its audit committee. There are two important points implicit in the question of where internal auditing will report: the level reported to must make the time to give serious consideration to the reports,[3] and reporting to the board implies that internal auditing does more than offer a service to the director—it provides a service to the board.[4] Both points must be evaluated by top management before any document is prepared defining the function's organizational status.

The second standard is that internal auditing should be able to communicate with the hospital's board. The Institute of Internal Auditors provides this standard to ensure that board members are kept informed. This line of communication also makes it clear to all hospital staff members that they should not interfere with the audit function. The applicability of this standard requires interpretation. The evolution of the boards of directors toward more interest and knowledge of hospital administrative affairs encourages the need for the director of internal auditing to keep the board informed of all significant findings. Board members or their audit committee, in turn, should take the time to consider the internal auditor's findings. To the extent the board is not prepared to deal with hospital management questions, the significance of the communication line diminishes. It is understandable, therefore, that the importance of reporting to the board will vary, depending on its composition and its level of participation in actually directing the hospital's administrative affairs. In any case, the independence of internal auditing will be enhanced if it is known that the board is informed of findings.

Third, the board should be notified in advance of a change in the director of internal auditing. Hospitals employing a staff of internal auditors will have a director. Hospitals with only one auditor may have an administrator fill the role of director, and the board should be kept informed of both the administrator's and auditor's employment status. It should be noted that an internal auditor working alone is capable of acting as the director of internal auditing in most cases.

Fourth, the board and hospital director must provide, in writing, a position description for the director of internal auditing, authorize access to all aspects of the institution, state the scope of the unit's activities, and define all reporting relationships for the function. The significance of this standard is clear. During the preparation of these statements, the administration and the director of internal auditing must be sure to meet the standards of the institute.

Fifth, the hospital director and governing board must be kept informed of all problems and limitations the internal auditing function is experiencing. Sixth and finally, all findings should appear in written reports to the board.

Another component of independence is objectivity. Objectivity for the internal auditor is composed of an attitude of independence, of not subordinating judgments on audit matters to others, of a belief in the unbiased nature of the work performed, and, last, of an unending pursuit of excellence in performance.[5] The internal auditor must be careful not to begin to see hospital activities in the same light as do department managers or the auditor will lose top management's perspective and the ability to evaluate critically a department being reviewed. The auditor must maintain a professional detachment from the area, its staff, and its management, while being careful not to alienate everyone. Personal biases for or against certain departments or managers can result in uncritical reporting or hypercritical head-hunting reporting. The important point is that human nature, lacking proper safeguards, can have an immediate negative impact on internal auditing's utility. It is only human to want to be liked by others, and in some cases to dislike others, as well as to be skeptical of reporting an adverse finding directly affecting a high-ranking administrator's area.[6]

To deal with human nature, the Institute of Internal Auditors has developed standards that place in the hands of the director of internal auditing the responsibility for maintaining objectivity. The director should assign work in areas where the auditor involved will have maximum opportunity to remain objective, and the director always must be alert for losses of staff objectivity. Items to be aware of in scheduling work are: not to allow a person who has worked recently in an area to audit that area, to rotate auditors on department audits, and not to allow an auditor to assume any regular operating responsibility. The problem of objectivity should be discussed during staff meetings and auditors should be encouraged to evaluate themselves critically and report instances when they believe they have lost objectivity.

The concept of rotating auditors has two implications deserving mention. First, rotating can cost money in terms of lost efficiency. The new auditor must become oriented and learn the new area. Second, rotating can save money because the new auditor, with a fresh perspective, may discover an important improvement consistently missed by the prior auditor. A rotation plan should be designed carefully to provide maximum gains.

One last point before concluding this discussion of objectivity: as noted, auditors must safeguard objectivity by not performing daily work or assuming responsibility for implementing changes within operating departments. It is only natural that an internal auditor probably would be less critical of systems and procedures that that individual had designed, implemented, and perhaps supervised. A dilemma quickly arises, however, when the management of the department audited is unable to respond to the needed changes because of managerial insufficiencies.

The internal auditor is responsible for reporting to the hospital director whether recommended changes, if agreed to, are implemented by the department's manager.[7] The extent to which an auditor can become involved with implementation without losing objectivity and without the hospital's losing the benefit of the proposed change is a question only the internal auditor can answer.[8] One possible method of dealing with the dilemma is to provide workshops to educate department managers enough to implement the change.[9,10] By taking this approach, the auditor will have provided management every available means of accomplishing the change without having assumed personal responsibility. The workshop approach would meet the criteria of the *Statement of Responsibilities* that adequate consideration be given and effective action be taken on all recommendations.[11] For many hospitals, even this approach may not be feasible, for management may be lacking in two respects in the department audited. First, the department may have no manager other than the best efforts of a senior employee or a secretary. Second, a manager may exist, but may be completely unequipped for the responsibilities of the role. The absence of effective management naturally is the root problem and must be reported to the hospital's director.

The question that arises next is whether the benefits of the change should be foregone until, or if, adequate management is acquired for the area. The answer must be no, and the responsibility may have to be shouldered by the internal auditor. Although assuming this responsibility definitely compromises objectivity, if internal auditing has enough employees and a shrewd director the impact of the compromise can be minimized by not permitting the auditor involved with the implementation to inspect the area in the future. For hospitals with few internal auditors, instances such as this will result eventually in management's absorption of internal auditing. The function must be safeguarded by the hospital director, although internal auditors may be called upon to change jobs and actually to join management.

To conclude, independence is important to internal auditing. Independence is achieved through proper organizational status and the pursuit of objectivity by all members of the internal auditing department. Loss of independence, to any degree, diminishes the usefulness of the function and should be watched over carefully not only by the director of internal auditing, but also by the hospital's administration.

SCOPE

The scope of internal auditing's work, as described in writing by the hospital director, should provide coverage for every aspect of the hospital's management and operation, without exception. Maximum service for the organization can be achieved only by allowing internal auditors to review and appraise every operation and its management. There seldom is an area run so perfectly that some improvement cannot be suggested and, in the rare instances when the area is perfect, confirmation of that fact is valuable.

The standards of the Institute of Internal Auditors cover four major areas that encompass essentially all operational and management aspects of any organization: (1) management information systems; (2) compliance with policies, plans, procedures, laws, and regulations; (3) economical and efficient use of resources and safeguarding of assets; and (4) adequacy of operating goals and objectives and the effectiveness of results.

Management Information Systems

Hospital directors depend on reports of operations for evaluation, control, and decision making. These reports often are inaccurate and may be unrepresentative because of poor design or because someone wishes to conceal ineffective performance. Even though hospital directors have a healthy respect for these reporting problems, they seldom have the time or expertise to appraise information systems. To have confidence in the information received, hospital directors must turn to the internal auditor for information validation. Internal auditors must be charged with the responsibility of determining whether all financial and operating reports are accurate, reliable, timely, complete, and useful and decide whether they are effective instruments for management control.

Compliance with Plans, Policies, Laws, and Regulations

The work environment of the hospital and its own environment are filled with policies, procedures, laws, and regulations too numerous to mention. Directors are responsible for ensuring that organizational participants and activities comply with hospital rules and with federal, state, and local laws. Directors must provide the means for compliance; internal auditors then must determine whether those means are sufficient and whether the institution is in compliance. Insufficient means and noncompliance should be spotted quickly, reported, and dealt with.

Use of Resources and Safeguarding of Assets

"Management is responsible for setting standards to measure operating performance and to establish controls over the use of resources and the safeguarding of assets."[12] The internal auditor learns whether adequate operating standards have been communicated by top management to everyone, and whether they provide accurate and timely measures of economy and efficiency. The internal auditor also must ascertain top management's reactions to reports of deviation from the control systems and the effectiveness of the responses for correcting the operating deficiencies. The auditor must appraise the overall effectiveness of control systems, for standards have little meaning without feedback as to whether they indeed have been met. The auditor is responsible for spotting conditions of idle or unproductive resources, unproductive work, costly procedures, and overstaffing and understaffing. The discovery of any of these conditions leads to a complete analysis of the control system's failure to provide management information on the waste.

Adequacy of Goals and Effectiveness of Results

How effective an organization is in meeting goals and objectives is essential to its continued existence. For private enterprise the ultimate goal is profit, while for the hospital it is outstanding patient care at a reasonable cost. Hospital directors must set the goals and objectives and establish an effective system of control to measure whether standards of performance that fulfill the goals and objectives are met. The role of the internal auditor in this important area is to ensure that goals and objectives have been set and that they are based on accurate assumptions and current and relevant information. The importance of auditors' reviewing standards, control systems, and corrective actions is apparent. Failure in any of these areas must be reported to top management, along with recommendations for action.

The scope of the internal auditor's work encompasses the entire hospital. The auditor must appraise all aspects of the top management's performance, as well as all management control systems. The adequacy of operating standards and the compliance of all members of the hospital (with policies, procedures, rules, and laws of both the institution and its social environment) must be reviewed. The scope of internal auditing is comprehensive. Without this scope, administrators would fail to gain the full insight the internal auditing function can provide into the entire hospital's performance. For the modern hospital, with its complexities and relatively independent operating units, the importance of this broad scope is critical.

PERFORMING THE MODERN INTERNAL AUDIT

While internal auditors appraise all aspects of top management's performance, top management itself must provide for standards and controls for the internal auditing function, as it would for other operating areas. Top management must be assured that all aspects of the direction and performance of audits are conducted with professional proficiency.

Managing Internal Auditing

The director of internal auditing is responsible for managing the function's resources effectively and for fulfilling the goals and objectives described in the operating statement of purpose, authority, and responsibility.

The director is responsible for all aspects of planning to meet agreed-upon goals and objectives. The director must prepare work schedules specifying what activities are audited and when and for how long. Scheduling takes into account such factors as when an area was audited last and the findings, changes that may be occurring, and potential loss risks. The director also must plan for staffing and for fiscal budgeting for the internal auditing function.

The director is responsible for preparing written policies and procedures to guide internal auditors. The extent of the procedures will depend on how many persons staff the function. A small number requires limited written policies and procedures because the director is in close contact with the staff. The director is responsible for developing written job descriptions, hiring, training, and evaluating personnel. Last, the director is responsible for a planned effort of assuring auditing quality. The director must evaluate all work continually for its manner of performance and provide for an annual review of overall plans with the hospital director and the governing board or audit committee. The director occasionally must arrange external reviews of the internal auditing function by qualified individuals.

Performing Internal Auditing with Proficiency

Performing an audit requires planning the activity; acquiring, examining, and evaluating information; communicating the results, and follow-up. Planning for an audit provides: (1) written objectives and scope for the audit; (2) acquiring general background information on the department; (3) informing managers concerned with the department's operations that the audit is to be performed; (4) conducting a preliminary survey to identify particular activities to review; (5) preparing a written audit program; and (6) identifying who should receive the report.

Departmental information must be collected and examined on all matters described in the audit's scope. Attention must be concentrated on collecting sufficient reliable information to support the audit's findings and recommendations. The end product will be working papers that document all findings and recommendations.

For the audit to be considered completed successfully, the results and recommendations must be communicated to all those having an interest in the department's performance. Before preparing a final report, the auditor should discuss the findings and recommendations with appropriate levels of management to gain acceptance of results and minimize misunderstandings.

The last phase of a successful audit is follow-up. The auditor should have a commitment from the department's management to implement the audit's recommendations, perhaps with a time schedule for the changes, or a clear statement as to why the recommendations were not accepted. After a reasonable time, the auditor should make a return visit to explore whether the recommendations have been adopted, whether they have been modified, and whether they are working. If necessary, the auditor may have to perform a brief reaudit to verify that the changes are working, with the results again reported to those concerned.

Professional proficiency is another important area affecting the overall utility of the internal auditing function. Both the director and individual auditors are responsible for professional proficiency. For example, the director should make every effort to assign to auditors work that they are prepared to handle, and auditors should decline work for which they do not believe themselves qualified. Ideally, there always will be an adequate number of qualified auditors, as a result of competent recruiting and selection of employees. Staff performance can be enhanced by programmed continuing education not only in technical areas but also in fields such as human relations and communications. Last, professional proficiency can be safeguarded by adequate supervision.

CONCLUSION

Board members, hospital directors and administrators, and internal auditors must understand what standards the internal auditing function must meet. Hospital managements have no one to blame but themselves if the internal auditing function is permitted to produce substandard results. Internal auditors will have no one to blame but themselves if their function fails to be accepted as a valued profession in the health care industry. Standards have been provided by the Institute of Internal Auditors that, when met, should produce outstanding results for the institution's board and director and earn the internal auditor an accepted niche in the hospital's management.

NOTES

1. T. E. Phillips, "Independence: Key to Successful Auditing—Both External and Internal," *Internal Auditor*, February 1978, p. 69.

2. The Institute of Internal Auditors, *Standards for the Professional Practice of Internal Auditing*

(Altamonte Springs, Florida: The Institute of Internal Auditors, Inc., May 1978), pp. 100–101.

3. Victor Z. Brink, James A. Cashin, and Herbert Witt, *Modern Internal Auditing: An Operational Approach* (New York: The Ronald Press Company, 1973), p. 31.

4. Victor Z. Brink and James A. Cashin, *Internal Auditing* (New York: The Ronald Press Company, 1958), p. 44.

5. The Institute of Internal Auditors, "Exposure Draft of the Standards for the Professional Practice of Internal Auditing," *Internal Auditor*, December 1977, p. 21.

6. Phillips, op. cit., pp. 68–74.

7. M. S. Armstrong, "An Auditor for the Seventies," *The Journal of Accountancy*, April 1976, p. 58.

8. D. Glass, "Results-Oriented Auditing and Independence," *Internal Auditor*, June 1975, p. 26.

9. B. E. Kaller, "Internal Audit: A Turnaround Situation," *Internal Auditor*, April 1975, p. 40.

10. J. Song and M. L. Carlson, "Improving the Internal Auditing Department," *Financial Executive*, October 1972, p. 37.

11. L. B. Sawyer, "What's the Internal Auditor's Responsibility for Corrective Action, Grandfather?" *Internal Auditor*, April 1974, p. 65.

12. The Institute of Internal Auditors, "Exposure Draft of Standards," p. 26.

Chapter 3

Internal Auditing Is for Hospitals

The fact that internal auditing is accepted by most industries and not by the health care industry is regrettable since it can play a very useful role in hospitals.[1] The function can benefit hospitals of all sizes regardless of whether it is available in the form of an internal auditing staff, as a staff shared with other hospitals, or by the use of existing staff members who have been trained to audit departments and functions other than their own. This chapter focuses on what hospital administrators and governing boards can and should expect from internal auditors.

The benefits hospitals can expect are the same as those that large corporations already experience. These include internal auditors:

1. appraising the soundness, adequacy, and application of accounting, financial, and operating internal controls, and promoting effective control at the least cost
2. appraising the extent to which employees comply with established hospital policies and procedures
3. appraising the accountability and safety of hospital assets
4. appraising the reliability of management information systems
5. appraising personnel performance
6. appraising all phases of management performance
7. recommending operating improvements

Internal auditors travel throughout the hospital, using a planned audit program. The result for all health care institutions will be improved efficiency and effectiveness, reduced risks and wastes, and improved operating controls and management information. No other staff function can accomplish such broad and demanding appraisals.

USING MANAGEMENT'S PERSPECTIVE TO EVALUATE MANAGEMENT INFORMATION

Internal auditors must have a firm grasp of hospital administrative functions and responsibilities and be able to place them in a perspective not only of the institution's management environment but also of its local, state, and national environments.

What should internal auditors be expected to know about hospital management? The more they can learn, the better. To evaluate the performance of even the simplest function, auditors must know how it should be performed, when, by whom, under what conditions, and with what expected result, and be able to relate the activity to a larger scheme of events. The internal auditor, to be fully prepared to analyze a function, must have a reasonably complete knowledge of how management would evaluate the function if it had the time. Failure to acquire an accurate management perspective will result in analyses and reports that fail to represent the administration's interest. A step beyond the operations analysis of a function occurs when the auditor actually evaluates management's role by asking questions such as: how was the function planned to perform and why, what goals and objectives were provided, has it been staffed properly, does it perform well, and does its service contribute to the hospital's goals? This evaluation assumes the perspective of the board of directors and the hospital director.

Internal auditors who have not acquired an educational background in hospital administration and have not sought diligently to learn about their institution's operations will experience limitations in fulfilling their responsibilities.[2] Auditors must read independently in general management and hospital administration to fill in missing background, and must continue to read to stay current.

The management process is considered by many experts to consist of planning, organizing, staffing, directing, and controlling. The process takes place in an environment filled with economics, technology, politics, social influences, and laws and regulations. The hospital also has many environmental factors that management must consider, such as limited resources, interpersonal and interdepartmental conflict and politics, and the many limitations human nature places on the best efforts of management to develop a rational organization in the institution.[3] As can be seen, the five management process attributes are carried on in an extremely large and complex environment, one that has become so large and complicated that many hospital administrators already have sought assistance from trained staffs of internal auditors.

Internal auditors, to be able to assist administrators in controlling the hospital, must be prepared to review all of the institution's activities with management perspective. One of the more important aspects of internal auditing is appraising the overall quality of the information management receives for use in performing its control function. "Perhaps the most basic problem the manager faces is the inadequacy of proper information."[4] If the information management receives through the formal reporting systems or from subordinates is unreliable, lacks essential facts, or is otherwise misleading, management works with less than perfect knowledge, and probably will not find out about a problem until it is too late.[5] If management cannot rely on what it sees or hears as being accurate and as fairly representing reality, how then can its information be validated as accurate? Other industries have found the answer in the internal auditing function.[6] Hospital administrators, before rushing out to advertise for a director of internal auditing, may wonder whether the information they receive is not reasonably accurate already. Perhaps it is accurate enough to get their job done. However, how would top management appraise its existing information to determine its accuracy? It would have to conduct a bottom-to-top review of all data gathering processes and of all processing to convert the data into meaningful summaries and reports, and closely examine the channels through which the reports are transmitted to the top. Such a review would take valuable management time that more than likely could not be spared from the continuing managerial process.

The problems all hospital administrators encounter with information are the result of the dysfunctions bureaucratic organizations have for twisting, bending, and concealing the truth. Social scientists have found employees are not likely to report their own failures to a superior. Departments also try to provide the best possible picture of themselves by taking calculated liberties with information, as well as by presenting management with exaggerated demands for more resources. A final problem results from lengthy communication channels—the longer the channel, the more likely distortion will occur. Distortion of this nature occurs with information going both up and down the hospital's organization.

The internal auditor breaks the cycle of questionable information flows by analyzing data gathering techniques and data processing procedures (whether manual or electronic) and by observing the information's flow to top management. Unsound and biasing procedures will be found and reported. As the auditor conducts the information appraisal, a second equally important assessment will be going on. Here enters the strongest application of the management perspective. The auditor must decide whether the information received by management, if accurate, is meaningful. Perhaps information is received routinely that is of no use to management, or is formatted poorly, or is untimely. Equally possible would be the discovery that important operational units of the hospital were providing inadequate or even no performance information to management. Regardless of the situation, the internal auditor has as a goal ensuring that top management receives accurate, timely, comprehensive, and meaningful information.

THE ROLE IN MANAGEMENT CONTROL SYSTEMS

Administrators are responsible for managing the hospital through internal control systems they specifically designed for their institution. The growth in hospitals' size and complexity has increased greatly the needs for and the demands on control systems. Internal control is the product of good managerial organization that provides constant measuring and evaluation of: (1) the representativeness and accuracy of data and reports, (2) the overall efficiency of the organization, and (3) the degree to which organizational participants follow policies and procedures.[7]

The nature of the control process encompasses seven steps.[8] First, top management must select and communicate the hospital's objectives. The entire staff should understand these objectives and, ideally, agree with them. Top management also should provide performance standards to guide all staff members on a job-to-job and day-to-day basis. Second, assuming the objectives have been stated in measurable terms, management must assess current performance. Third, performance results then must be compared with the objectives. Fourth, causes for variance above or below the objectives must be analyzed. Fifth, top management must determine what corrective action is in order. It must make two basic managerial decisions: after searching for the causes of the variance and determining possible avenues for improvement, it may decide (1) the objective cannot be reached and lower it, or raise it if performance has been above expectation; or (2) management may choose a course of action to solve the problem and continue to seek to fulfill the objective. Sixth, management must implement the new course of action and take the time to supervise it. And seventh, the results of the new action must be reappraised constantly, based on the measurement of results.

It is apparent from this that top management control depends on effective planning, organization, staffing, and directing.[9,10] Control is an attribute of the management process that can function meaningfully only if the administration has provided the hospital with an effective process. A failure in any part of the management process can have a negative impact on both the performance and uses of control. Controls may become ineffective when hospitals are organized or staffed improperly. Personnel may not know to whom to report variances and middle management may be uncertain about who is responsible for directing the area in question. Lack of planning and development of objectives and performance standards may make the best of control systems ineffective because there is nothing to which results can be compared.

Good control systems do not just happen, they must be developed painstakingly, and even after they are established they must be supervised constantly. The internal auditor has an important role in ensuring that top management has provided a good control system and in assuring the administration the system is working well. The auditor must:

- determine whether management has provided adequately defined and measurable objectives and that the objectives are realistic and oriented toward the control of the most important resources and activities of the hospital
- explore the nature of the control system to determine whether the measurement processes are accurate and timely and place reports of performance results into the right hands and, in instances of variances, see to it that the administration responds to the reports.

Internal auditors can fulfill this function for the hospital because of their professional expertise, independence, and objectivity. They rely on an understanding of general management and hospital administration and the ability to cross and recross operational areas while tracking down all components of control systems. The ability to evaluate findings objectively is the internal auditors' key contribution in evaluating hospital control systems.

INTERNAL AUDITING AND COST SAVINGS

Administrators of hospitals without internal auditing, while perhaps recognizing the value of the function, may believe the added expense is not justifiable. Internal auditing's track record in industry should dispel any reservation about its ability to earn its way. The function is suited ideally to proving itself in health care institutions:

1. Internal auditors serve the hospital by acting as an extension of management. In doing so, they identify and report problems. They do more than search and report; they recommend improvements. Depending on the numbers and types of problems they encounter, they may present many cost savings and income-generating recommendations for management's consideration.

2. Most of the 7,000 health care establishments in the United States receive an annual visit from a certified public accounting firm. The amount of work the firm performs depends in part on how adequate a hospital's internal control is, especially in fiscal matters, and the professionalism of the internal auditing function. Internal auditors have as a goal ensuring that good internal control has been established over the institution's assets and its accounting and financial reporting. The amount of review a CPA firm will have to perform is related directly to the adequacy of the controls. Sound internal control will reduce the total time and cost of a CPA engage-

ment by 10 to 15 percent.[11] More savings are available if the CPA personnel work with the internal auditors by allowing the latter to perform many of the routine, time-consuming tasks—a common practice where the CPA firm's personnel perceive the internal auditing department to be independent.

3. A good internal auditing operation is a training ground for hospital administrators. The function provides a unique opportunity to learn in detail the operations of all the institution's departments and activities.[12,13] The internal auditing unit may suffer to some degree if its personnel constantly are promoted to administrative posts. A possible solution is to rotate administration members through internal auditing on an annual basis. There is one positive benefit of cannibalizing the internal auditing department for administrators: senior auditors may become less productive because of slowly acquired conflicts with some departments or because of tendencies to show their power, so a maximum service life for an auditor may be appropriate.[14] Auditors may be changed to administrative positions where their insights into the hospital's operations may be used well.

CONCLUSION

Hospital administrators must have a solid understanding of internal auditing before they can develop a need that requires filling. Internal auditors have the important responsibility of performing all their duties with excellence and with a scope that provides outstanding service to the institutions that employ them. It is through this sharing of knowledge about internal auditing and through documentation of service to hospitals that internal auditing will spread gradually throughout the health care industry. Wherever there are hospitals large enough to rely on formal bureaucratic organization structures that distort information and make effective management control difficult, there will be a need for internal auditing.

NOTES

1. R. S. Smith, "Why Not Internal Auditing?" *Hospital Progress*, January 1968, p. 56.

2. A. E. Marien, "Why Have Internal Auditing?" *Hospital Financial Management*, December 1969, pp. 28–29.

3. W. Burns, "What Top Management Expects of Internal Auditing Now!" *Internal Auditor*, June 1975, p. 17.

4. Victor Z. Brink, James A. Cashin, and Herbert Witt, *Modern Internal Auditing: An Operational Approach* (New York: The Ronald Press Company, 1973), p. 48.

5. S. D. Watson, "Internal Auditing Viewed from the Top," *Internal Auditor*, December 1973, p. 29.

6. "Internal Auditing: A Primer," *Hospital Financial Management*, June 1975, p. 43.

7. Victor Z. Brink and James A. Cashin, *Internal Auditing* (New York: The Ronald Press Company, 1958), p. 10.

8. Victor Z. Brink, James A. Cashin, and Herbert Witt, pp. 58–60.

9. L. G. Pointer, "Internal Auditing Comes of Age," *Internal Auditor*, October 1973, p. 38.

10. C. L. Kampmann, "Internal Control Is for Management, Too," *Hospital Financial Management*, September 1970, p. 15.

11. E. H. Fly, "Cut Your Auditing Costs by Auditing," *Hospital Financial Management*, December 1968, p. 13.

12. The Institute of Internal Auditors, *Promoting Professional Progress* (New York: The Institute of Internal Auditors, Inc., 1956), p. 73.

13. Burns, op. cit., p. 18.

14. J. Song and M. L. Carlson, "Improving the Internal Auditing Department," *Financial Executive*, October 1972, p. 36.

Chapter 4

The Operations Auditing Approach

Operations auditing is the most recent and potentially useful development of internal auditing. Operations auditing has been mentioned briefly earlier. It is time now to examine this new approach in detail. Hospitals will gain maximum benefits from internal audits conducted with the operations approach. While financial and compliance auditing will continue to play a role in health care institutions, major improvements in patient care and cost containment will be produced by operations audits. Operations auditing, as noted in Chapter 1, has not matured to the point of having a definition suitable to all practitioners. This epitomizes the evolving nature of this type of auditing. Operations auditing is reaching out to encompass the total spectrum of management and organizational behavior and, since management science and behavioral science continue on the march, so must exponents of operations auditing. Whatever the ultimate form time holds for operations auditing, it has something to contribute to hospitals. This chapter introduces the basic elements of operations auditing and relates them to the hospital environment and the administrator's daily management responsibilities. It also highlights the important areas of operations auditing for hospital internal auditors.

OPERATIONS AUDITING'S NATURE

The lack of an acceptable definition of operations auditing leads naturally to a listing of some of the more enlightened attempts to describe it:

- "As a representative of administration, the internal auditor investigates and determines whether or not departments have a clear understanding of hospital and departmental objectives, whether they maintain proper records, whether they accurately record, protect and manage: cash, inventories, equipment, supplies and personnel and how they interact with other departments in the hospital."[1]

29

- "Operational auditing is an activity which is concerned with the examination and evaluation of management and its operational controls, and is made with the purpose of formulating recommendations that will lead to increased operating efficiency."[2]
- "Operations auditing is a technique for regularly and systematically appraising unit or function effectiveness against corporate and industry standards by utilizing personnel who are not specialists in the area of study with the objectives of assuring a given management that its aims are being carried out and/or identifying conditions capable of being improved."[3]
- "Basically, an operational audit comprises an analytical survey of business activities to determine their adequacies so as to achieve managerial policies and objectives and to establish the degree of adherence to the prescribed system."[4]
- "A rather common misconception on the part of some internal auditors is that there is a clear-cut distinction between operational auditing and traditional financial auditing. Auditors look for special manuals which will tell them how to make operational audits when all that is really necessary is a change in their own manner of approach and analysis. The narrow type of internal auditing will be largely directed to protective analysis and appraisals, often in relation to some set of dogmatic standards of financial control. Operational auditing begins with familiarization with actual operations and operating problems, followed by analysis and appraisal of the controls to assure that they are adequate to protect the business."[5]

THE OPERATIONS AUDIT

The Institute of Internal Auditors' *Standards for the Professional Practice of Internal Auditing* (Appendix A) recommends four steps that apply to operations auditing:

1. planning the audit
2. examining and evaluating information
3. communicating results
4. follow-up

Planning the Audit

The first three stages of planning include: (1) reviewing all background information about the department to be audited, and (2) establishing preliminary objectives and scope for the work.[6] Objectives and scope may be provided by the director of internal auditing or worked out in conjunction with departmental management and the auditor assigned the task. The objectives and scope must act as guides and not as inhibitors. Once these steps are complete, (3) the department and all interested administrators should be informed and permitted to discuss the audit.

The next major step generally is referred to as familiarization with the department's objectives, how work is organized and performed to accomplish the objectives, and how results are determined.[7] Familiarization begins with an in-depth discussion with the department manager. The auditor should learn:

1. the exact function and operative activities of the department
2. the organizational relationship of the area to the rest of the hospital
3. problems the department encounters in achieving its objectives and any plans for change
4. policies and procedures for the department, which should be available in written form; if not, the auditor should request they be prepared in writing as they are crucial in determining standards of performance
5. an understanding of the department's operations, which should be discussed with other department managers and supervisors to find out if everyone knows the objectives, policies, and procedures and to check the accuracy of the auditor's perceptions; information based on hands-on work experience often will be volunteered and frequently will provide key insights into the department's daily performance
6. the physical lay-out of the department, which should be inspected to help tie together all that has been learned during interviews; during the inspection, the auditor should be alert for safety hazards, employee work habits, the condition of the plant and equipment, actual work organization, security, and anything of further interest

The importance of familiarization cannot be overstressed. The auditor must know what is being done, how it is being done, why, and whether it contributes to the hospital's objectives.[8]

The final step of the planning process is the preparation of a written audit program. The program should state the objectives and scope of the audit and provide a detailed outline of all the steps expected to be taken. The program should be approved by the director of internal auditing or a suitable representative of management.

Examining and Evaluating Information

Once all planning steps are completed, the auditor starts the fact-gathering process based on the audit program. The auditor may use any of a large number of statistical testing and sampling techniques to examine records and to evaluate information provided to management. The auditor will document and record all findings carefully on specially designed worksheets. The emphasis of this portion of the audit is on collecting information, with strict attention to every detail of documentation. The auditor will make recommendations for improvements based on these findings. To the degree the auditor fails in fact gathering and documenting, the individual becomes increasingly more vulnerable to embarrassing revelations and counterassertions based on more credible documentation by the department's management. To avoid these difficulties, the auditor must be sure to have acquired sufficient, competent, relevant, and useful information: sufficient in the sense that it be factual, adequate, and convincing; competent in the sense of reliable, best, and most timely; relevant in the sense that it supports findings and recommendations; and useful in the sense of again supporting findings and recommendations, but also in terms of benefiting the hospital.

One of the biggest pitfalls in gathering information is loss of objectivity. The auditor may become obsessed with proving a point of view to the exclusion of other equally useful information that does not support the individual's opinions. A second pitfall is an instance when department management presents the auditor with plausible but undocumentable explanations for deviations from expected performance. For example, the author witnessed a fruitless effort by an auditor to prove or disprove the effects of sex, weather, and holidays on the food consumption of dormitory dining rooms on a large college campus.

The auditor is completely dependent on knowing the facts and interpreting them correctly. Work in the department must be exhaustive and must be reviewed by the director of internal auditing; it is recommended that findings be discussed with other colleagues. A new perspective may develop suddenly that dramatically alters the interpretation of some information. During and after the fact-gathering process, the auditor should communicate findings and results to all members of management concerned with the department reviewed.

Communicating Results

An audit involves two levels of communication—informal and formal. The informal involves discussions and interim written reports. The informal communications often deal with obtaining the department management's interpretation of findings and its acceptance of various recommendations. Problems that produce immediate losses and inefficiencies should be brought to the department manager's attention for prompt correction. The overall tone of these communications should be aimed at gathering management's support and interest. A byproduct of the audit work and discussions should be the education of department heads about the meaning of internal auditing as a management service in the hope that audits will not be perceived as threatening.

A highly recommended communication step is the submission of a preliminary draft of the report to the department's management, followed by a meeting to discuss the report.[9] Department managers should be permitted a final opportunity to present their points of view before the report is issued. The internal auditor's presentations during the meeting should be directed at packaging and selling recommendations to make them most acceptable to the department managers. The final product of communication is agreement on operating changes needed to improve efficiency and achieve objectives. Instances when agreement is not achieved should be noted in the formal written report.

The second level of communication is formal. The auditor prepares a written report of all findings, recommendations, and opinions and distributes it to a predetermined list of managers and administrators. Accepted rules of report writing should be observed and adequate supporting documentation provided. The administrator or manager directly responsible for the area should respond in writing, with particular attention to actions that will be taken on recommendations.

Follow-Up

Internal auditing's responsibility does not end with reporting. The auditor must prepare a schedule for follow-up visits to determine whether departmental management has implemented the changes agreed to and, briefly, to appraise their effectiveness. Depending on what is found, further action may be necessary. Unfortunately, not all managers are cooperative and skilled in implementing changes, and all the recommendations may not solve the problem. The auditor is responsible for keeping both the department head and the hospital director informed of instances of poor management response at the departmental level.

PRACTICING HUMAN RELATIONS IN OPERATIONS AUDITING

In reviewing the structural elements of an operations audit, the need for the auditor to practice good human relations is evident. The auditor usually will be regarded as an outsider and all too frequently as threatening. Employees may conspire actively to conceal operating problems, or they may work with the auditor on a passive-aggressive basis. The auditor must make a reasonable effort to dispel employees' fears and anxieties and solicit their assistance.

The internal auditor experiences built-in problems and resistance that arise from employee fears that the results will cause them to be punished by management.[10] This negative image results from the almost policelike activity of financial and compliance auditing in the past. Employees might be familiar with other types of audits, such as those of the Internal Revenue Service, that further aggravate their anxiety.

The internal auditor, then, has a special mission in performing an operations audit. These fears and anxieties, which often lead to resistance, must be dealt with successfully. One book suggests the most effective approach is to seek to develop a partnership relationship:

> This partnership approach emphasizes the common interest of both the auditor and the auditee to join with other company personnel to find more efficient and more effective ways to carry out all types of operational activities. It is this common interest which makes it possible to subordinate individual personal interests, and to find a bond which can be the basis of good cooperation and productive results.[11]

A second factor that will help to create a better image is an outstanding job.[12] Few elements work more quickly to establish the acceptance of operations auditing than the development of outstanding findings and recommendations that will enable all employees to perform their work better.

No one formula will work for all auditors all the time. The internal auditor must be sensitive to the managers and employees whose work is being reviewed.[13] In the hospital, this responsibility is even more significant because of the many professional personnel involved. The director or administrator of internal auditing should visit departments routinely after projects are completed to gain some sense of how the employees feel about the audit and auditor. An auditor who arouses ill feelings fails the test of professionalism, regardless of the adequacy of the findings and recommendations.

CONCLUSION

Operations auditing is the most valuable tool the internal auditor has to offer hospitals. Through this approach the entire hospital will be audited. The performance of operations audits is based on well-established principles that, when combined with a successful human relations approach, yield a wide assortment of findings and recommendations for improvement that department managers will accept and implement willingly.

SUMMARY OF PART I

This chapter concludes discussion of the foundations of internal auditing and their applicability to the health care industry. These foundations will apply to all the remaining chapters, which have as their purpose developing a framework for the use of modern internal auditing in hospitals.

NOTES

1. R. N. Gilbert, "Operational Auditing," *Hospital Financial Management*, August 1977, p. 30.

2. C. T. Norgaard, "Operational Auditing: A Part of the Central Process," *Management Accounting*, March 1972, p. 25.

3. Roy A. Lindberg and Theodore Cohn, *Operations Auditing* (New York: American Management Association, 1972), p. 9.

4. R. S. Polimeni, "The Operational Auditing of Quality Control," *Internal Auditor*, February 1975, p. 39.

5. Bradford Cadmus, *Operational Auditing Handbook* (New York: The Institute of Internal Auditors, Inc., 1964), p. 9.

6. Victor Z. Brink, James A. Cashin, and Herbert Witt, *Modern Internal Auditing: An Operational Approach* (New York: The Ronald Press Company, 1973), p. 100.

7. Cadmus, op. cit., p. 25.

8. Ibid., p. 26.

9. E. H. Fly, "Cut Your Auditing Costs by Auditing," *Hospital Financial Management*, December 1968, p. 14.

10. L. E. Berry, "Are You a Thick-Skinned Auditor?" *Internal Auditor*, February 1976, p. 44.

11. Brink, op. cit., pp. 114–115.

12. Xerox Corporation, "Internal Auditors: People Who Lend a Helping Hand," *Internal Auditing*, February 1977, p. 26.

13. W. J. Harmeyer, "Some of My Best Friends Are Auditors But . . . ," *Internal Auditor*, February 1973, p. 10.

Part II

Developing Internal Auditing in Hospitals

Chapter 5

Starting Internal Auditing

Chapters 1 through 4 dealt with internal and operations auditing concepts but not how hospital administrators and internal auditors should go about setting up an effective function. Chapters 5 and 6 fill some of the void by presenting an outline for starting internal auditing, anchored in preparing the hospital for the function and recruiting a qualified person to direct the program. Governing boards and hospital administrators must be committed to establishing an internal auditing program and prepared to support it with resources and a suitable organizational environment.

Hospital administrators planning to start such a program first should contact the local chapter of the Institute of Internal Auditors. The institute fully supports the concept of progress through sharing. Local chapter members will be likely to volunteer time to educate administrators, to assist them in developing a basic business organization for internal auditing, to design the basic charter for the function, and to write a job description for the new director. Another helpful source is the certified public accounting firm employed by the hospital. That firm usually will have employees capable of guiding hospital administrators through all phases of developing an internal auditing capability.

The second step is to recruit an individual capable of doing an excellent job of managing the function and carrying it out, as would be the case of smaller hospitals where one auditor would be enough. Once the right person is hired, the hospital's top management and the new auditor must develop a close working relationship to define the scope and independence of the function and prepare an operating manual.

The auditor must gain firm support from top management and the governing board. The auditor in larger hospitals also must learn whether more resources will be allocated to the function to nourish its growth. If substantial support is promised, there is a definite need to prepare plans for organization and management of the function and job descriptions for the rest of the staff.

Hospitals that have internal auditing should review these chapters to determine whether their current operations are in compliance with the guidelines presented.

RECRUITING A LEADER FOR INTERNAL AUDITING

Hospitals of 250 beds will find a full-time auditor of benefit.[1] Hospitals of 500 beds or more should be considering two or more auditors with supporting clerical and secretarial staff. Smaller hospitals with less than 250 beds can share a staff of internal auditors with other nearby hospitals or hire an auditor who also may have to act as manager of a department in the hospital.[2] The important point is that all hospitals, at some time, may recruit an internal auditor. Although only one person may be hired, that individual should be a good leader and manager as well as a good practitioner. Hospital directors must make every effort to recruit a person who will be outstanding in terms of leadership, integrity, and professional competence. An internal auditor without the goals of personal and professional excellence will not contribute to the hospital's performance in the manner exemplified by many of the better auditing departments in other industries. The responsibilities of internal auditing are much too important to entrust to a person who does not believe in excellence.

What attributes help to identify an outstanding applicant for internal auditor? There are two basic categories: professional ability and character.

Professional Ability

Professional ability may be dealt with best by dividing it into education and training, work experience, and special certifications. Most experts believe the person responsible for the overall internal auditing program in a hospital should have a strong accounting and finance background. This translates to a bachelor of science degree in accounting. Some contend that of equal importance is an educational background in business administration or hospital administration, which translates to a master's degree in business or hospital administration. An MBA with a background in accounting and finance is recommended for director of internal auditing. Some courses in the humanities and behavioral sciences are needed. Familiarity with statistical sampling and electronic data processing also is important.

Work experience is the melting pot for educational background. Candidates should be able to demonstrate they have a strong work background in management and internal auditing acquired principally in corporations or other industries, but with some experience in hospitals. Beyond the accounting background, hospital management experience may have to have been gained as an assistant to an institution's controller or financial executive. This background will be beneficial because of the hands-on experience with hospital accounting and finance. Experience as an internal auditor may well have had to take place outside of the health care field because of the low level of development of the function in hospitals to date. This is not a serious problem so long as the applicant has worked for a company with a sound internal auditing department. The field of internal auditing is so universal that a good auditor will acclimate quickly to the health care industry.

Specialized certification programs are a popular means of guaranteeing that a certain basic level of professional competence has been achieved. There are two types of certification: as a Certified Public Accountant (CPA) or as a Certified Internal Auditor (CIA). CPAs are certified by states and usually are required to have a certain minimum number of years of accounting practice. Applicants with CPA certification also should have several years of responsible work experience in industry. The second and new form of certification, the CIA, has emerged from programs sponsored by the Institute of Internal Auditors. Certification in one or the other is preferred as an indicator of academic and work achievement.

Character

A person's character is a combination of qualities or attributes that distinguishes that individual from all others. Successful internal auditors have many attributes that distinguish them from less acceptable candidates. Some of these attributes are:

- Adaptability. Internal auditors must be adaptable to meet the demands of shifting constantly from one audit and department to another. Internal auditors are faced with a constant learning process that is more stressful than the jobs of department managers, who learn their function but once.
- Understanding. Internal auditors must be able to understand human motivations and failures. They must have compassion for top management and department administrators when problems are found.
- Determination. Internal auditors must be determined to get answers to all their questions, to explore all exceptions found until their causes are known, and to press forward in the face of difficulty and opposition when making recommendations.
- Creativity. Internal auditors must be creative and resourceful when designing audit programs, when carrying out the programs, and when making recommendations for changes.
- Versatility. Internal auditors must be able to move constantly from one audit to the next without losing their ability and enthusiasm for appraising each department's operation.

- Integrity. Internal auditors always must be certain to not compromise their code of ethics, their goal of aiding the hospital as a whole, and their responsibility for professional performance of their duties.
- Alertness. Internal auditors always must be alert for operating problems and improvements.
- Tactfulness. Internal auditors must be able to approach top and middle management with problems that are found and recommendations for improvement without arousing defensiveness and hostility.
- Helpfulness. Internal auditors always must have an attitude of trying to help the management of the area they are reviewing.
- Good communication skills. Internal auditors must be able to communicate effectively with top and middle management and with colleagues.
- Self-assuredness and rugged individualism. Internal auditors are subjected to many personal pressures in their roles as appraisers of performance. They must not give up in the face of opposition and criticism.
- Willingness to get involved. Internal auditors must identify with the hospital and its goals, believe in its mission, and seek through auditing to help it to fulfill its mission to society.

Recruiting the leader for the internal auditing function is an important step. It may be surmised from the education and work experience requirements that applicants will be in their mid-thirties or older, with seven to ten years of work experience. Hospitals recruiting more than one internal auditor will be able to lower the requirements for hiring the balance of the staff. The most important point that bears reemphasis is that all hospitals recruiting internal auditors should hire as their first individual, even if it is to be their only one, a person of outstanding leadership and professional ability.

CONSOLIDATING TOP MANAGEMENT'S SUPPORT

The new auditor, hereafter referred to as the director of internal auditing, must acquire, if not already available, a comprehensive written directive or charter from the hospital's top management that provides sufficient scope, independence, access, and authority for the performance of the function. The preparation of the charter should be based on Chapter 2 and the new *Standards for the Professional Practice of Internal Auditing* (Appendix A).

Of equal importance, the director must acquire top management's support. Operations auditing cannot be productive unless it receives solid endorsement from the top.[3] This means more than enfranchising the function; it means solid backing as resistance and criticism are encountered. Internal auditors, especially while conducting operations audits, are not likely to tackle really tough problems and issues if they do not believe top management firmly supports their efforts. The director of internal auditing must seek constantly to develop ever better rapport with top management to ensure the proper level of backing is present and, if possible, improved upon. This will entail a campaign to sell the administration on the new function.[4] Naturally, the sales job will succeed only if internal auditing is attracting substantial positive attention by performing competently and professionally. Success at gaining top management's support may be measured by the actual backing received when difficult problems arise, and from the expansion of the function through the administration's allocating more resources to its performance.

ORGANIZING THE INTERNAL AUDITING FUNCTION

The director of internal auditing should work with top management to develop a detailed operations auditing manual. The form and content of the written policies and procedures should be appropriate to the size and structure of the function and the complexity of its work.[5] An audit staff of one or two persons probably will have only a small manual; however, development of operating problems may be a good indication that written policies and procedures covering at least the basic standards of performance should be prepared. Administrators of hospitals large enough eventually to employ a full staff of internal auditors should work with the director of the unit in preparing a manual to avoid crisis situations as the number of auditors reaches critical mass and informal management techniques break down.

A typical manual will include: (1) guides for performance that ensure adequate coverage and quality; (2) administrative procedures that guarantee smooth running; and (3) daily operating instructions.

Guides for Performance

There are many possible performance guides. Below are 12 subjects the manuals should cover that will help auditors consistently to carry out programs that meet the standards established by the director of internal auditing and the hospital's top management:[6]

1. The objectives of the audit should be defined clearly to avoid the temptation of exploring unplanned operating areas outside the department being audited.
2. The service the audit will provide must be determined. What will the audit accomplish? Will it be restricted to a narrow review of one sus-

pected activity or will it encompass the entire function and its relationship to the rest of the hospital?

3. The scope of the audit usually will cover all operations of a department. What activities, methods, procedures, and operating objectives will be examined? Are lines of authority and responsibility documented?

4. The customary steps of a preliminary review must be provided. Old audit reports should be read, recent literature reviewed, and the hospital's written directives for the department studied.

5. The format of the preliminary discussions with the department's management on the audit's objectives and approach require documenting. Guides to timing and the various management levels to be involved should be provided.

6. The manner of conducting the preliminary survey and the information to be obtained must be explained.

7. The requirements that must be met when preparing the written audit program must be presented in detail. The audit program will guide the remainder of the project, must be complete and concise, and must adhere to established objectives and scope.

8. The auditor's responsibility for completing work within the budgeted time must be discussed completely.

9. Standards for all workpapers and documentation must be provided in detail.

10. Policies for reporting preliminary findings and discussing suggested changes with management must be provided.

11. Guidelines for preparation of written reports are an absolute necessity.

12. Instructions for replying to department managers' responses to the report recommendations must be available to guide the auditor during follow-up to ensure corrective action has been taken.

Administrative Procedures

Every staff function or similar department should establish instructions (preferably written) for daily operations. For the internal auditing function there are four basic subject areas: office administration, personnel, audit projects, and audit reports.[7] Office administration should cover filing systems, supplies, time reports, correspondence, and reporting. Personnel procedures should include personnel records, travel instructions, evaluations, and reports of absence, sickness, or injury. Under audit projects are such topics as assigning work, human relations, time budgets, requests for audit program revisions, uses of statistical sampling, safeguarding workpapers, and interviews with management to conclude the audit. Audit reports may involve the use of interim reports, supervision of report preparation, and proofreading and report distribution.

Daily Operating Instructions

Thus far this volume has dealt with matters that, once written, will change slowly. This is not true of daily operating instructions. The instructions may be communicated formally or informally and may or may not be in writing. Because of their nature, the director of internal auditing must make a continuing effort to keep an up-to-date record of all of the more important daily instructions issued. No listing will be provided here of the more frequent types of daily instructions. The need for and types of such instructions will depend on the organizational climate of the internal auditing function and the quality of the auditing staff. Nothing will wilt morale more quickly than conflicting and possibly discriminatory instructions that, when put to the test by the staff, appear arbitrary because of lack of documentation and purposeful planning by the director.

One last important aspect of organizing the function is the preparation of job descriptions for all internal auditing staff members. This step should be taken even in hospitals where the function is performed only on a part-time basis. Even in the largest hospitals, the director should be able to supervise all staff members. Therefore, other than the requirements for the director's position, there need be only one other general type of job description into which can be fitted persons with specialized backgrounds in EDP, accounting, finance, and operations auditing. Separate job descriptions for secretarial and clerical supporting personnel should not be written if the hospital already has suitable ones available.

Examples of job descriptions for full-time positions of director and auditor are provided below.[8] Part-time position descriptions may be evolved from the full-time ones to suit the needs of small hospitals.

The Director of Internal Auditing

General Responsibilities

The director of internal auditing is authorized to direct a comprehensive program of internal auditing within the hospital. Internal auditing will examine and evaluate all activities as to the adequacy and effectiveness of management and its contribution to the goals of the hospital. The internal auditing function is authorized unrestricted access to all hospital activities, facilities, and records.

Specific Responsibilities

1. prepare an operating manual and direct work through the guides for performance, administrative procedures, and daily operating instruction
2. develop an audit program to evaluate the hospital's management control system
3. prepare a comprehensive, long-range program for audit coverage

4. examine all departments and levels of management for compliance with hospital and departmental policies and procedures
5. make recommendations for improving management control and information systems and department operation
6. review and appraise procedures, records, policies, and plans of departments audited to ensure they accomplish their intended objectives
7. authorize the release of audit reports
8. appraise the adequacy of middle management's response to correct deficiencies cited
9. conduct special reviews requested by the administration
10. coordinate the internal auditing program with activities of the hospital's CPA firm and various other auditors representing third-party payers such as Medicare

Supervisory Responsibilities

1. supervise the work of all auditors and support staff
2. assign budgets of staff hours for completion of audits and develop a schedule to control audits
3. review work to determine whether it meets the standards for performance
4. review and approve the preparation of all audit programs

Auditor

General Responsibilities

1. perform assigned work
2. evaluate the adequacy and effectiveness of the administration's management control-system
3. determine the extent operating units and personnel perform work in compliance with hospital policies and procedures
4. plan and perform work in accordance to standards established by the director, including verifying and analyzing transactions and the preparation of work papers
5. prepare reports of all findings and provide recommendations for improvements

Specific Duties

(performed under the general guidance of the director)

1. survey assigned functions to learn about operations and assess the adequacy of management control and information systems
2. determine scope and objectives of the audit

3. prepare the audit program with emphasis on clearly describing the various auditing techniques to be used and the key points in the area to which they will be applied
4. perform the audit in a professional manner
5. appraise the adequacy of the corrective measures taken by middle management

Supervisory Responsibilities

1. supervise auditor assigned to the audit

Much hard work is required of the director and top management to establish a firm basis for organizing and managing the internal auditing function. Even though the amount of work will vary a great deal depending on the hospital's size, it is extremely important to do a good job on the tasks required by the hospital's size and staffing requirements. Without these building blocks, the internal auditing function's contribution in terms of improving a hospital's operation will be restricted unnecessarily.

CONCLUSION

Hospital directors who plan to develop an internal auditing capability have a major responsibility for recruiting a person with outstanding credentials and skills as the leader of the new function. Top management must be prepared to stand behind internal auditors as findings are developed and recommendations made that may produce new pressures on the managers of various departments. Top management and the director of internal auditing must work together to develop the basic charter for the performance of the new function's organization and control. Chapter 6 continues this discussion by providing guidelines for selecting and training the auditing staff.

NOTES

1. E. H. Fly, "Cut Your Auditing Costs by Auditing," *Hospital Financial Management*, December 1968, p. 15.

2. Ibid, p. 15.

3. Roy A. Lindberg and Theodore Cohn, *Operations Auditing* (New York: American Management Association, 1972), p. 22.

4. Lawrence B. Sawyer, *The Practice of Modern Internal Auditing* (Orlando, Fla.: The Institute of Internal Auditors, Inc., 1973), p. 20.

5. The Institute of Internal Auditors, *Standards for the Professional Practice of Internal Auditing* (Orlando, Fla.: The Institute of Internal Auditors, Inc., May, 1978), pp. 500–503.

6. Sawyer, op. cit., pp. 14–16.

7. Ibid, pp. 16–17.

8. Ibid, pp. 8–13.

Chapter 6

Selecting and Training an Internal Auditing Staff

Recruiting a good leader and practitioner as the director of internal auditing is the most important step in developing a highly useful function. Directors of hospitals large enough to employ a staff of two or more auditors should apply many of the same criteria and methods of selection for the other positions as those used in identifying the director of internal auditing.

The first section of this chapter more fully develops the recruiting and selection process as it applies to hiring a staff of auditors. The second section discusses the means and methods of keeping internal auditing staffs current on theory and practice. Directors of hospitals that have internal auditors, or eventually will recruit them, will want to be assured that their staff is kept up to date through the mechanisms of continuing education and in-house training programs. Managers of hospitals employing only one auditor should be certain to encourage that individual to keep current and, from time to time, discuss progress on continuing education and training. A highly qualified staff of internal auditors who are exposed constantly to new education and training will be prepared to provide an outstanding service to the hospital.

RECRUITING AND SELECTING STAFF AUDITORS

Recruitment of auditors may take place both within the hospital and outside of it. Internal recruiting has the advantages that applicants are familiar with the health care industry and the specific institution and their performance, character, and personality are better known.[1] A further advantage may accrue when the person, after several years as an auditor, returns to manage a department in the hospital. Already mentioned is the fact that experience gained from auditing many areas of the hospital provides outstanding training for future administrators.[2] A negative aspect of internal recruiting is that applicants may lack a broad background from working in different industries and different hospitals. Should qualified in-house applicants be lacking, outside recruiting will be needed. Good sources of candidates are college and university departments of business, hospital administration, and accounting. The fact that many opportunities exist for springboarding from internal auditing into management is a good basis for selling college graduates on internal auditing. A second source of outside candidates is certified public accountants who may be looking for a change in career direction. Advertisements in accounting journals and large city newspapers within a 200-mile radius will produce many qualified applicants. Another source is internal auditors from other industries who may be reached by advertising in *The Internal Auditor*.

Once a pool of good candidates is available, the selection process begins. This will entail interviewing and possibly testing.

The interviews should be conducted in an organized manner using commonly accepted methods. The interviewer will be interested in sizing up the candidate and selling the individual on internal auditing. The same character attributes listed in Chapter 5 are applicable to recruiting staff auditors. The person's personality, appearance, and presentation are important. Immediately afterward, the interviewer should record all impressions received and any information acquired that was not on the employment application and résumé.

It is important to sell candidates on careers in auditing and point out the professional development opportunities available. The new meaning of modern internal and operations auditing often is not known by candidates. Applicants may visualize auditors as wearing green eyeshades and spending an exhaustive amount of time in financial and compliance work.[3,4,5] Time must be spent explaining the role and scope of internal auditing, and answering questions. It is advisable to have a job description and related literature on hand to give to applicants.

The use of testing in selecting internal auditors is debatable. The process is tied inseparably to test validation or the degree to which tests predict performance. One author suggests there are three possible areas on which to test candidates: (1) writing ability; (2) ability to organize thoughts; and (3) ability to differentiate between fact and conjecture.[6] A fourth area of importance is clerical skill. Should the director of internal auditing want to explore possible uses of testing, it is recommended qualified assistance be sought from the hospital's personnel manager and possibly a consultant. Testing must be approached with great care. Excellent candidates may be dismissed from consideration because of poor performance on a section of the test that, in fact, does not predict performance.

STAFF DEVELOPMENT

From the first hour of employment, the auditor should be subjected to a planned program of personal and professional development. The first phase is an enlightening employee orientation program. This will set at ease the new auditor's concerns over being comfortable in the job and being accepted by the organization and its staff. Disillusionment and a loss of motivation can occur quickly if the orientation is not planned and structured carefully. Much thought should be given to orientation, and written guidelines should be prepared. The limited internal auditing staffs in smaller hospitals generally will require the director of internal auditing to play a strong role. An orientation manual or booklet may be written and given to each new employee. The manual should provide a brief history of the hospital, the internal auditing function, and general rules of work such as hours, vacation policies, and so on. General guidelines for work performance and evaluation also can be provided. The director should introduce the new auditor to the staff and other key individuals in the institution. A walk-through of the hospital also is in order.

The importance of a well-planned staff development program including both internal and external training cannot be overemphasized. Internal auditing is a rapidly evolving profession that requires a constant level of continued training to stay current. Four broad areas for training and continuing education can be planned:[7]

1. familiarization with hospital, departmental, and internal auditing policies and procedures
2. professional training in such areas as typical hospital operating problems, basic supervision of employees and auditors, human relations, and report writing
3. specialized professional training in electronic data processing, finance, social insurance regulation, and advanced management analysis techniques
4. personal and professional development, often using college campuses or Institute of Internal Auditors or American Management Association seminars on such subjects as general management principles, economics of health care, laws and legislation, and social responsibility

Each of these areas requires in-depth consideration and will have to be tailored to the hospital's needs and the audit staff's size and levels of training. Once the content, direction, and emphasis of the staff development and training program is decided on, the training methods must be chosen. The most common ones can be grouped into four general categories:

1. On-the-job training probably is the best method when the employee is working with a skilled auditor.[8] The new auditor can be guided carefully through many learning experiences and permitted to complete selected work with a minimum of supervision. Care must be taken to not compro-

mise this valuable training method by pressing new auditors into assuming responsibilities for which they are not prepared but may be willing to try to handle. On-the-job training is suited especially for the familiarization phase of learning auditing and hospital policies and procedures.

2. Individual study of professional journals and literature, manuals for internal auditing, and other materials such as hospital and departmental manuals covering the broad scope of the institution's operations, while closely related to familiarization, may be regarded as a second important source of knowledge. Auditors must take the initiative to improve themselves. Much can be learned from journals on hospital management, financial management, and internal auditing. Specialized training manuals often are available that can educate the auditor on such topics as uses of statistical sampling and inventory and personnel management. Manuals prepared by the director of internal auditing for that function and by top management for department directors should be studied carefully. Well-prepared operating manuals can provide the auditor with many insights into auditing the hospital and how the administration believes the institution is or should be operating.

3. In-house staff training meetings are a third commonly used method. Staff training meetings can be very productive if planned properly. Training program topics may include the internal auditing organization's administrative rules and regulations; changes occurring in the hospital; specialized training in, for example, statistical sampling; and previously assigned research topics.[9] An important benefit of these meetings unrelated to training is that they provide a forum for discussing procedures, salary and wages, promotions, and other problems. The director must be careful, however, not to allow the meetings to lose their training benefits by permitting too much discussion of staff problems and disagreements with policies.

4. Formal classroom training, such as special seminars sponsored by outside professional organizations, class attendance on a college campus, or enrollment in correspondence courses, is an important ingredient of any program. Although taking advantage of these opportunities requires the expenditure of funds by the hospital or the employee and the loss of working time, much is to be gained by such a formal approach to staff development. The classroom provides many opportunities to learn the newest auditing and hospital management techniques and to acquire education in specialized areas such as auditing electronic data processing. New perspectives may be gained that will lead to more innovative solutions to old and unresolved hospital operating problems. It is important to discuss the costs of this type of training. Costs for employees to attend seminars and college courses and the time lost from productive auditing are less real than they

seem at first. When it is considered that in-house training has costs in that the director or someone else must prepare the materials for training meetings and that auditing time will be lost while attending the sessions, the expense of outside training becomes relatively less.

It is the director's responsibility to organize and control the use of these training techniques. Attention must be given to providing a proper mix of all four to provide the best opportunities without losing sight of cost effectiveness. An intangible benefit of a good training program is improved morale and enhanced ability to retain auditors longer.

CONCLUSION

One of the most important investments of time and money a hospital and internal auditing director can make is in a comprehensive, well-planned, and well-executed training program for staff auditors. Administrators of hospitals too small to employ more than one auditor must assure themselves the auditor is seeking and receiving continued training.

Hospitals large enough to require two or more auditors must be sure to make available to the auditing staff financial and time resources to pursue advanced education and training.

SUMMARY OF PART II

This chapter concludes the discussion of the practical steps required to set up an internal auditing function in a hospital. Once internal auditors are hired and ready to start work, problems of managing and coordinating the various audits must be handled. Coverage throughout the hospital must be planned and directed skillfully to gain the maximum service internal auditing has to offer. After planning comes the actual performance of the audit based on many time-tested internal auditing techniques. Chapters 7 through 9 will present actual internal auditing as it is practiced in hospitals.

NOTES

1. Victor Z. Brink, James A. Cashin, and Herbert Witt, *Modern Internal Auditing: An Operational Approach* (New York: The Ronald Press Company, 1973), p. 596.

2. B. E. Kaller, "Internal Audit: A Turnaround Situation," *Internal Auditor*, April 1975, p. 37.

3. Roy A. Lindberg and Theodore Cohn, *Operations Auditing* (New York: American Management Association, 1972), p. 31.

4. J. R. Deters, "Renovation and Innovation in Internal Auditing," *Internal Auditor*, June 1975, pp. 30–31.

5. A. W. White, "The Essentials of an Effective Internal Audit Department," *Internal Auditor*, April 1976, pp. 30–31.

6. Lawrence B. Sawyer, *The Practice of Modern Internal Auditing* (Orlando, Fla.: The Institute of Internal Auditors, Inc., 1973), p. 31.

7. Brink, op. cit., p. 600.

8. Lindberg, op. cit., p. 31.

9. Sawyer, op. cit., pp. 56–57.

Part III

The Practice of Internal Auditing in Hospitals

Chapter 7

Long-Range Planning for Maximum Benefits

Chapters 5 and 6 covered the how-to of building an internal auditing function without offering guidelines on exactly how to manage it once a staff is employed and ready to go. The next three chapters provide the basic framework for planning, directing, and controlling the function from the point of view of hospital directors and directors of auditing programs. Hospital directors must have a complete understanding of this framework to be able to evaluate internal auditing's performance. They must be familiar with the principles of effective audit program management to be certain internal auditing's full potential is realized. The first and most basic management component is planning. Careful planning of where, what, how long, and how frequently to audit ensures the best possible coverage of all hospital departments with a frequency and audit intensity selected to utilize best the available resources.[1]

PREPARING STRATEGIC PLANNING WITH MANAGEMENT

The new director of internal auditing as well as those who have been on the job a few years can benefit from involving the hospital's top management in planning the overall strategy of audit coverage. Top management and the internal auditing head must be certain that the planned coverage includes all of the hospital's major management problems and most of the routine operating issues.[2] The planning period should cover two years in detail and may be extended to five years in general outline form.[3,4] The period for detailed planning must allow for at least one audit of all departments, even if some may have to be audited every third or fourth year because of a lack of staff. Strategic planning should concentrate on the worst problem areas with the greatest exposures and risks, explore known weaknesses of departments and of systems that span departments, target management levels where corrections must originate, and evaluate the availability of resources and the expected cost effectiveness of the audits planned.[5] Top management involvement is imperative in order to surface the important problems and issues and gain management's perspective of them.

An important related benefit of involving top management in planning is that the expected role internal auditing is to play in the hospital becomes much clearer to top management as the plans are prepared. The director of internal auditing should not miss the excellent opportunity planning meetings provide to sell internal auditing. A management thus sold will be much more receptive to and supportive of audit report findings and recommendations.

The planning process must not create a system to be served. While providing control and structure, planning must not produce restrictions and rigidity. Provision must be made for changes of direction as needed and for special assignments; however, care must be taken that plans not be abandoned in favor of industrious fire fighting.

Once a strategic plan has been agreed to by top management and the director of internal auditing, the outline and all supporting ideas should be assembled into a formal document that will be used as a benchmark for evaluating progress. The internal auditing head then must use the plan's framework to allocate resources and coordinate individual audits with the activities of the departments to be inspected.

PREPARING A STAFF-HOUR UTILIZATION BUDGET

A good staff-hour utilization budget is an important step in the planning process. The budget requires assigning particular personnel for each project for each year and allocating a set number of hours for each audit. The starting point for preparing the budget is to list all planned audits down the left side of a page and a five-year period across the top. The strategic planning process has provided the director of internal auditing with the frequency and intensity of each audit and the frequency that unplanned special reviews may be requested. Based on this information, the audit frequency can be written after the title of each project and the best auditor for the job assigned. The director then must estimate the number of hours required for each audit and enter the figure under each year the project is to be performed. Once the worksheet is completed, the total number of hours for each year and each auditor can be added and compared with the total number of hours available in the year less expected absences such as for vacation, illness, and planned training.

Budgeted hours per auditor may be adjusted if too few or too many hours had been planned originally. The director may have to reduce the time initially planned for some audits to lower the total hours to match the staff hours available or add hours or projects if too few hours were assigned initially. The director also may have to reassign audits to different staff members if an auditor's hours still are oversubscribed. The purpose of estimating the hours for each audit is to provide perspective when the available staff-hour resources are considered. The director of internal auditing may conclude that the function is overstaffed or understaffed or does not have the right mix of talent. Hospitals should not lose sight of what resources ideally should be available to fulfill the function best.

A last point is that staff-hour budget planning forms an important quantitative basis for personnel evaluation. For this reason the staff-hour budget should be posted, each audit's budget discussed with the auditor, and written procedures developed for modifications. These changes should be agreed to in writing and the plan amended accordingly.

COORDINATING AUDIT COVERAGE

This is the final phase of the planning process. Strategic planning produced an audit strategy of where, how often, and with what intensity audits should be conducted. Staff-hour budget planning provided who and how long. The coordinating process is concerned with when. When is the best time to visit a department in terms of being least disruptive? When is the best time relative to the planning and change processes of the hospital as a whole? When in terms of other audits that may impact on the department or activity to be reviewed? And when in terms of the audit program? Well-organized coordination is essential to ensure that the long-run cumulative impact of audits and reports is favorable and that unnecessary inconveniencies are not imposed on audited departments.

When for the Department

Auditors must try to fit audit schedules to the affected department's expected workloads.[6] All departments have some peaking of workload throughout the day, week, month, and year. The director of internal auditing should visit the department manager to ascertain the nature of the unit's workload. A particular time of the year may be better than another, or a particular day or two in the week, or particular hours of each day. Once this is determined, the director and the auditor assigned can plan the project for the most convenient times and either perform work that does not require being in the department or carry out other audits during the peak workload periods. This consideration for the audited department will demonstrate the professional approach of a good internal auditor and surely will win friends in the unit.

When for Hospital Planning and Change

There seldom is anything more disheartening to the auditor than to labor long and hard only to discover the hospital is planning or soon will implement changes in the department. This essentially nullifies the part of the audit affected by the changes. It also wastes time. If the auditor had been aware of the changes, the program very likely would have been modified to assess their impact on the department and its problems. The director of internal auditing should be kept informed of all of the hospital's planning and decision making. The hospital administrator responsible for the department should be interviewed before starting the audit to be certain there are no plans or changes of which the internal auditing head and the auditor are not aware. Knowledge of the type, extent, and timing of changes will enable the auditor to adjust the program to provide the most useful analyses of the proposals. This may mean abbreviating the audit to concentrate on spotting problems and returning after the change has been implemented to find out what affect it had on them.

Some departments may be found to be in a chronic state of change. This often occurs because of frequent shifts in a department's management, in its resources, in its operating environment, and in operating procedures such as the adding of computer capabilities or the rewriting of computer programs. Determining whether the changes have solved the problems often has to be postponed for an extended period until the rate of change slows or stops. The auditor, when confronted with this circumstance, is encouraged to meet with the hospital administrator in charge of the department and the department's manager to discuss the planning behind the changes. The auditor may observe deficiencies in the planning and implementation that seriously compromise their usefulness.

When for Audits of Related Areas

The benefits of this form of coordination are observed easily but are difficult to achieve. An audit of ordering, receiving, and warehousing will play a role in evaluating the absence or overabundance of supplies in departments. An audit of the personnel budgeting process will provide information for evaluating findings of overstaffing and understaffing in departments. This aspect of coordination is subject to a great deal of perfecting. The director of internal auditing at all times must be aware of changes in audit programs and the addition of special projects. Many of the problems of coordination can be anticipated; however, many can be learned only from experience while trying to coordinate audits with crossover effects. The best time to adjust previously prepared plans for this type of coordination problem experienced during audits is after each audit is completed. The director can review the project as completed and try to fit it better into the overall audit program.

When in Terms of the Audit Program

The scope and purpose of the audit must not be changed too much from the original strategic planning process. The audit program requires certain steps to be executed in a prescribed order and often at a predetermined time. It may be necessary to observe activities as they are performed. The audit program may require the review of a day's or a week's work immediately after the period ends. Equally possible, the audit program may be performed at only one time in a year, such as an annual inventory of supplies and equipment before the end of the fiscal period. Regardless of the exact nature of the audit program's restrictions, all such curbs must be weighed against the three other coordination elements, and a harmony must be found.

Coordinating internal audit coverage fine-tunes the use of staff-hour resources to provide maximum results. It is important for the hospital director to review the internal auditing chief's efforts toward improved coordination and the auditing head must keep the hospital manager informed of changes in strategic planning produced by efforts at coordination.

CONCLUSION

The creation of an overall audit program strategy with large contributions from hospital and internal auditing directors is crucial in determining the eventual utility of the function. All phases of detailed planning such as the generation of staff-hour budgets and coordination of audit coverage must be discussed with hospital directors to foster additional input and to keep communication lines open and functioning. Hospital and internal auditing directors must be committed to making time for proper planning.

NOTES

1. Victor Z. Brink, James A. Cashin, and Herbert Witt, *Modern Internal Auditing: An Operational Approach* (New York: The Ronald Press Company, 1973), pp. 578–580.

2. L. B. Sawyer, "Professionalism in Internal Auditing," *Internal Auditor*, February 1976, p. 19.

3. Ibid., p. 18.

4. A. E. Marien, "The Internal Auditor Manages through an Audit Program for a Hospital—Part I," *Hospital Financial Management*, December 1968, p. 34.

5. W. A. Tuthill, Jr., "Managing the Audit Functions: A Formidable Challenge," *Internal Auditor*, June 1974, pp. 23–24.

6. Roy A. Lindberg and Theodore Cohn, *Operations Auditing* (New York: American Management Association, 1972), p. 23.

Chapter 8

Standard Internal Auditing Techniques

With the planning processes completed, auditing can begin. The director of internal auditing has selected the auditor best suited to perform the work based on education, ability, and prior experience. The director and auditor now must meet to discuss the instructions for the project and the time budget. After receiving instructions, the auditor proceeds to acquire a working knowledge of the department to be reviewed by reading literature on its activities and past audit reports and by visiting the unit. Based on what is learned, the auditor designs an audit program tailored to provide a thorough review of the department that will meet the standards established by the instructions for the project. With the program in hand, the auditor examines the reports, documents, and data that compose the audit trail. Once the fieldwork is completed, the audit report is prepared. The report is the final and most important step of an audit and most of Chapter 9 is devoted to a complete explanation of the reporting process.

PREPARING AUDIT INSTRUCTIONS

The number of instructions needed for an audit will depend on its size and complexity and the auditor assigned. While the total may vary, there are at least eight specific areas that instructions should cover:[1]

1. The nature and scope of the audit must be described clearly, and objectives set that, if met, will fulfill the planned scope.
2. The director of internal auditing may have acquired special insights and information that bear on the project. The department may have a unique organizational structure, unusual interrelationships with other departments, a leader with an unusual personality, or particular problems that have been extremely persistent.
3. The scope of discussions with management must be defined, particularly what levels of management will be interviewed and to what extent. An

important point, previously mentioned, is that all hospital plans and operating changes affecting the department must be ascertained.

4. The availability of department manuals on procedures and activities should be discussed and their possible uses in the audit described.

5. The operational relationship of the auditor with the department's personnel should be stipulated. The auditor has no authority over such personnel and must safeguard independence and objectivity by not becoming personally involved with the unit's operation.

6. The reporting requirements for the audit must be agreed on, and the need for oral and written interim and final reports and the personnel to receive them should be discussed.

7. Procedures must be provided if hazardous situations for patients, employees, and the hospital are discovered or if potentially illegal behavior is uncovered.

8. The audit's time budget, its possible revision, and other assigned personnel must be discussed in detail and preferably be summarized in writing to avoid any misunderstandings as to expectations and timing.

The manner of conveying the instructions is important. Written instructions, if well prepared, leave little room for doubt in the event the auditor fails to follow them but they take time to write and type and may make the process of instructing the auditor unnecessarily formal and impersonal. It is recommended a complete discussion of all instructions be held with the auditor, who is given an opportunity to question them. Once the instructions have been conveyed verbally, understood, and agreed to by the auditor, at least instructions one and eight should be put into writing. It is the director of internal auditing's responsibility to tailor the instructions to fit the needs of both the audit and the auditor.

PERFORMING THE PRELIMINARY SURVEY

The audit program's design must be based on the most accurate and complete information available. The program forms the basis for the execution of the audit and its accuracy is as essential as the accuracy of blueprints for a building.

The preliminary survey begins with the auditor's researching materials available in the auditing office. If the department has been audited previously, that file should be examined. All findings, recommendations, correspondence, audit report replies, and notes should be read. A summary of important points should be made as starting places for checking. Other materials such as hospital and departmental manuals and hospital policies and procedures that apply to the department should be studied. For additional perspective and insight, the auditor should obtain published articles or books on the department or its type of work.

Based on this research, the auditor can prepare a list of questions to learn more about the department and fill in knowledge gaps. It may be advisable to prepare a formal questionnaire and submit it to the manager to obtain even more information.[2] Internal auditing literature provides many lists of questions that may be compiled into a questionnaire. A good questionnaire often can surface problems of which management is not aware and guide the auditor to the preparation of a better program.[3] The objective of the preliminary survey is to avoid wasting time and perhaps becoming hopelessly mired in activities and issues of little importance. The auditor must have a clear idea of what information is needed.[4]

The auditor now is prepared to schedule the introductory meeting with the department manager. Sufficient time to cover all the questions should be requested. The first meeting should be limited to two hours, preferably between 9 a.m. and noon.

The auditor should be familiar with typical interviewing techniques and approach this first meeting with a cooperative, friendly attitude that will develop rapport with the manager.[5]

That the auditor has prepared for the meeting and knows something about the department will help the manager develop confidence in the questioner. The first meeting is an opportune time to educate the manager about internal auditing in general, explain the nature of the assignment, and answer questions. The goal of this introductory portion of the meeting is to set the manager's mind at ease and begin to gain the individual's confidence. The auditor next must begin the information-gathering process. Listed below are examples of some of the more common questions.[6,7] The auditor should select the more important ones to be answered first, leaving the less important ones for future meetings.

General Operating Information

1. Ask the manager to describe the mission of the department. Encourage the manager to "tell it like it is" and not recite a statement from a policy manual. Inquire what basic activities carry out the mission.
2. Request an up-to-date organization chart and relate the department to the hospital's overall organization chart. Inquire about the department's interrelationships with other hospital departments. Fill in on the chart the names of assistant managers and supervisors and the numbers of persons under them.
3. Review fiscal and budget information to gain more perspective on the size of the department and the hospital resources involved. Observe the location and manner of retention of fiscal and budget data.
4. Obtain a copy of operating instructions and manuals not covered during the office research phase.

5. Ask the manager about particularly bothersome problems that have proved difficult to solve.
6. Prepare flow charts of management information flows and other pertinent paper trails as needed. The extent of flow charting will depend on the size and complexity of the department.
7. Accompany the manager on a walk through the department. Be sure to see all the space the department controls. Make general observations as to the physical condition of the department and its equipment, ask for brief overviews of systems and procedures, discuss and observe activities performed, and observe employees at work.
8. Inquire about plans for change and about any modifications about to be made or recently implemented.

Planning

One of the principle products of planning is the creation of guiding objectives and the setting of goals that will help fulfill those objectives. Below are some important questions to be answered:

1. Have objectives been established for the department?
2. Have they been stated formally?
3. Are the objectives in agreement with those of the hospital?
4. How were they established, when, and who participated?
5. Are the objectives realistic? Are there enough resources available and are there any external constraints?
6. Are the objectives set high or do they foster mediocrity?
7. Do the goals motivate personnel to extend themselves?
8. Are the goals measurable and have criteria been established for evaluation?
9. Are objectives and goals reevaluated periodically?
10. Do reports accurately and fairly represent performance?
11. Are specific persons identified as responsible for accomplishing goals and have the goals and objectives been communicated clearly to them and all employees?

Organizing

Properly organized work activities help to integrate the total work effort of the hospital. Below are questions that must be explored to determine the degree to which all management levels have accomplished this important and difficult task.

1. Have all the department's resources been placed in a structural relationship with each other that promotes achieving the objectives?
2. Are resources available in the right quantities at the right place and time?
3. Does the organization promote continuity and the assumption and discharge of responsibility?
4. How rigorously is the department organized? Does everyone know what to do, when and where?
5. How often is the organizational structure reviewed?

Controlling

Good internal controls over all phases of work is a necessity for top management in order to determine the degree departments have not previously agreed to objectives. Below are questions which must be answered.

1. Have standards of performance been set and are there good measurement methods? Is there evidence that management responds to failures?
2. Are employees properly trained for their jobs?
3. Are there systems of internal checks?
4. What records are available and how are they maintained?
5. What feedback exists from other departments on interrelationships?
6. Do employees understand the department's objectives and goals and do they know and follow instructions?
7. What routine management monitoring processes exist?

Staffing

Hospitals must be properly staffed to be able to render quality health care at reasonable costs. Below are questions which will examine the staffing arrangements of hospitals.

1. Are the employees qualified for their jobs?
2. What efforts are made to train them further?
3. Is there evidence of good personnel administration of matters such as reporting time, illness, vacation; do job descriptions exist; is there much turnover?
4. Do employees appear to be motivated and interested in doing a good job?
5. What appears to be the quality of supervision?

All of these points obviously cannot be covered in a two-hour meeting. The auditor will need to return to the manager many times to become fully familiar with the department. A recommended procedure is to close the meeting with the physical inspection of the department's spaces and be introduced to all assistant managers and supervisors. Many questions can be answered by the assistants— in some cases, more accurately and completely. Most of the points apply to all areas and must be answered before the audit program can be designed. A good preliminary survey ensures an intelligent audit examination, and many times part of the survey may substitute for the detailed examinations required by the program.[8]

PREPARING THE AUDIT PROGRAM

The audit program is a carefully designed plan for detailed analyses of fiscal and operational activities. The design should demonstrate the auditor was well informed about the department and approached the project with innovativeness and imagination.

There are two basic types of audit programs that may be used in hospitals. The first is one that, once designed and perfected, will not be expected to change much from audit to audit. It is presumed the department also will change little from audit to audit and that the subject matter lends itself to this type of treatment. Examples of such areas are handling of cash, investments, accounting, and certain purchasing elements such as receiving. The use of preprepared audit programs provides improved coverage of routine areas with the added benefit that findings are comparable between locations and from one report to the next.

The second type of audit program is the individualized plan designed specifically to fit the auditor's interests or theories for the project and the department's unique characteristics. The auditor, after completing the preliminary survey, will have decided that some basic operating activities, procedures, and management problems are of particular interest.[9] These interests will become the core of the audit's theme or theory.[10]

The key to the audit program's design is to incorporate a thorough review of the objectives of the department with an evaluation of their achievement.[11] It must not be forgotten that the role of the internal auditor is to provide a review as though top management were conducting it. Top management would appraise the achievement of objectives and assess their contribution to the hospital's overall performance. The auditor must accomplish this evaluation or expect a less than enthusiastic response to the final report.

The audit program also has an impact on managing the project. With all the steps of the audit formally organized and listed and with specific techniques decided on, time and personnel allocations can be made. The auditor in charge will have little difficulty keeping effective control of a large or complicated project by using the program as a management control device.[12] The audit program also forms an objective basis for requesting more or less time for the project and for changes in direction.

The audit program must be written immediately after completion of the preliminary survey while all ideas and details are fresh in the auditor's mind.[13] The auditor must not do a rush job of designing a program. The design is subject to a great deal of perfecting. The final draft should be presented to the director of internal auditing for evaluation. Once a program design is agreed on, it must be discussed with the department manager to keep that individual informed and to encourage feedback on points overlooked or not emphasized enough in the project.

The actual preparation of audit programs cannot be dealt with in detail here. Preprepared and individualized programs will cover every conceivable aspect of a hospital's operation and management. Further, they may be designed from almost any perspective, based on each auditor's own abilities and theories. There exists a considerable pool of information on audit programs. Even though many audit programs found in books, manuals, and periodicals were written for other industries, many can be adapted to the health care industry. The *Internal Auditor* frequently has material on audit program design. Journals of related fields such as certified public accounting often have detailed discussions of audit programs that can be adapted. Finally, the Institute of Internal Auditors or the hospital's CPA firm may be contacted. CPA firms have resources at their disposal that may be shared with hospital internal auditors. Hospitals sponsored by the federal government, armed forces, and states, if not visited routinely by auditors from central offices, often can obtain assistance from them.

A sound program will make an average auditor look good and a good auditor look outstanding. Although specific information on audit programs cannot be provided, six points can be reemphasized as crucial to all such projects:

1. The auditor must know the program's planned scope and objectives.
2. The auditor must know exactly what the department's objectives and goals are and how they relate to the hospital.
3. The auditor must know the information flows that make up the department's system of management control and reporting.
4. The auditor must know the time budget and the number of other persons assigned to the audit.
5. The auditor must know the hospital's exposure in the department to loss or risk and its impact on patient care.
6. The audit program must not become an end in itself. It must not restrict the inquiring mind of a good internal auditor.

FOLLOWING THE AUDIT TRAIL: THE FIELD WORK

Field work basically is a process of measurement and evaluation.[14] The auditor must measure and evaluate all activities in the department.

Measurement

The auditor must decide what to measure and to what degree. The what is determined by the department's activities and the availability of an audit trail. In many cases there will be paper flows that produce documentation of performance. In such instances, the auditor must choose the extent of detail of the measurement. If the department has good internal checks and balances and is not judged to be a high risk area, a minimum of measuring may occur. A survey or sampling may suffice. The higher the risk and the fewer the number of internal checks and balances, the greater the need for in-depth and detailed data gathering. There will be instances where what is measured is not nicely documented by paper flows; in such cases, the auditor should recommend that the department develop documentation in the future. Where documentation is lacking, the auditor must be innovative and resourceful in trying to measure the activities. Measurement may take the form of interviews and observation, as might be the case with a poorly documented planning or organizing process.

Measurement generally takes six forms in internal auditing:[15]

1. The auditor must be a keen observer of everything that takes place in the department. The auditor will have made many observations during the preliminary survey, but observation must continue throughout the program. The auditor must be aware constantly of seeing and hearing things that are not indicative of a well-managed hospital department. The auditor may observe a wide range of unacceptable items such as lack of cleanliness, safety violations, wasted employee time, unused or broken equipment, poor planning and control, and major problems in patient care.

2. The auditor must become an artful questioner. Skillful questioning often can lead to the discovery of operating problems the audit trail otherwise might not uncover. Employees may volunteer subjective information that, when added to other findings, points to problems not anticipated originally. In some instances, interviews may be the only means of gathering information. The auditor must be effective in obtaining information through questions and not create an atmosphere of cross-examination that will provoke a defensive response by employees.

3. The auditor must be good at analyzing the information thus gathered. Much of it will have been organized on worksheets designed to facilitate analysis of the data. The auditor wants to uncover causes and effects and must reassess the audit's methodology continually to be certain no operational elements are missed. The auditor may discover a certain sequence of events that requires an in-depth analysis before conclusions can be drawn as to the quality of performance.

4. The auditor must verify the accuracy of data gathered, the representativeness of employee statements, and the accuracy and meaningfulness of man-

agement information. The auditor must be certain that statements made in the report are supported by factual data and information.

5. The auditor also must be adept at investigation. The auditor frequently will be confronted with events that require careful scrutiny and systematically must track down evidence on a particular problem, whether it be an impropriety or an instance of mismanagement. An investigation may arise as part of an audit or be assigned as a management request. The auditor must be careful to not become too involved in criminal investigation. After spotting apparently illegal activity, the auditor should leave the actual investigation to hospital security and local police, but remain available should the auditor's skills be needed in analyzing records.

6. An important tool that is being perfected and applied in an ever larger number of internal audits is statistical sampling. This should be used to examine a series of many transactions. Proper application of statistical sampling can yield excellent information in a minimum of time. Internal auditors must be prepared to use the method wherever possible. A great deal of literature, as well as seminars, is available from the Institute of Internal Auditors to help guide the auditor in using statistical sampling.

Evaluation

The second element of following the audit trail is the evaluation of findings. Evaluation requires professional judgment and comparisons with standards.

The auditor first should evaluate the adequacy of established standards for hospital performance and, where they are lacking, request that they be established. The auditor may decide that existing standards are ambiguous or set too low relative to the individual's conception of an absolute standard or as compared with the industry's standards. The auditor may discover that standards set long ago no longer apply and need revision. The auditor assumes an active role in assuring that the hospital fulfills its objectives, and must evaluate the standards before applying them to operations.

The auditor must compare all findings with standards of performance established by top management to determine the adequacy of the department's efforts. The auditor's findings should be assembled in a format that makes this comparison as straightforward as possible. Judgment and opinion should not be involved if at all possible. The auditor must be capable of evaluating deviations from standards and develop recommendations for improvement where standards have not been met. Instances where standards have been exceeded also should be reviewed. The department may have concentrated on some activities to the exclusion of meeting standards for others. The standards may have to be revised upward, the better to reflect performance capabilities.

CONCLUSION

The evaluation of the audit findings concludes the field work. The auditor now is ready to assemble all of the worksheets, documentation, and recommendations and write the audit report. The report is the final product of all the hard work and will be only as good as the effort put into the preliminary survey, the audit program, and the field work. However, an outstanding audit can be compromised completely by a poorly prepared final report ignored by top management and department heads. Chapter 9 provides many of the principles of writing an audit report that will ensure management acts on it.

NOTES

1. Victor Z. Brink, James A. Cashin, and Herbert Witt, *Modern Internal Auditing: An Operational Approach* (New York: The Ronald Press Company, 1973), p. 607.

2. F. T. Carlin, "Operational Auditing and the Questionnaire," *Internal Auditor*, October 1975, pp. 69–75.

3. A. E. Marien, "An Internal Control Questionnaire for a Hospital," *Hospital Financial Management*, March 1969, pp. 32–34.

4. Lawrence B. Sawyer, *The Practice of Modern Internal Auditing* (Orlando, Fla.: The Institute of Internal Auditors, Inc., 1973), p. 127.

5. W. J. Harmeyer and R. A. Wood, "Audit Interview Techniques, a Behavioral Approach," *Internal Auditor*, February 1975, pp. 13–22.

6. Dale L. Flesher, *Operations Auditing in Hospitals* (Lexington, Mass.: Lexington Books, 1976), pp. 36–38.

7. Sawyer, op. cit., pp. 135–149.

8. Ibid., p. 124.

9. Bradford Cadmus, *Operational Auditing Handbook* (New York: The Institute of Internal Auditors, Inc., 1964), p. 33.

10. Sawyer, op. cit., p. 155.

11. Ibid., p. 157.

12. M. A. Dittenhoffer, "The New Audit Standards and Internal Auditing," *Internal Auditor*, February 1974, p. 18.

13. Sawyer, op. cit., p. 165.

14. Ibid., p. 274.

15. Ibid., pp. 283–289.

Chapter 9

Audit Report Preparation for Management Action

The written report of the audit's findings, corrective actions, and recommendations is the internal auditing function's direct link with the hospital's top management. The internal audit report must catch top management's attention and imagination by providing clear, concise statements of findings, actions agreed to and implemented by department managers, and carefully designed and documented recommendations. The report must be oriented for management action. The entire audit will have failed in its objective if the administration fails to respond to its recommendations.

Preparation of a report aimed at management action begins with the working papers. Properly prepared and organized working papers make the writing of the audit report much simpler. Reporting involves meeting standard report-writing criteria; use of proper formats, style and editing; reviewing preliminary drafts with the internal auditing director and the department's management, and formally presenting the report to department heads and top management. Submission of the report does not conclude the audit. The department's management must respond in writing and state actions it will take on the audit's findings and recommendations. The last step is to follow up on whether management actually took the agreed-upon actions and that they solved the problems.

WORKING PAPERS

Working papers must accomplish a number of functions if they are to serve their purpose effectively.

1. Thoughtfully prepared, designed, and organized work papers are of great assistance in carrying out the audit's field work in an orderly manner. At a glance they show the audit's progress, problems encountered, and any weaknesses of the program's design.

2. Working papers are a record of work done and a repository for findings.[1,2] As a record, they help the auditor manage and control what at times amounts to a vast array of information, findings, and problems. As a repository they become important as a source of documentation for deficiencies and recommendations for change. Finally, the papers form an important basis for supervision of the auditor and evaluation of performance.[3]

3. Working papers are the foundation for writing the audit report and for all interim reports and discussions.[4] They assist the auditor in locating deficiencies, assessing performance, and arriving at conclusions and recommendations. Working papers are the ultimate source for documenting findings and recommendations and frequently will be called upon to defend the auditor and the report. Last, the working papers facilitate report writing. At times the auditor will be able simply to summarize and rephrase many of the statements in the working papers as the report is written.

4. Working papers become historical documents.[5] Months after completing the project the auditor may have to turn to them to answer a question posed by top management or to help departmental management solve a persistent problem. Years later the working papers will be consulted by those assigned to reaudit the department.

The value of carefully designed and organized working papers cannot be understated. There are a number of practical steps for creating highly useful working papers.

1. During the preparation of working papers, the auditor must be sure to keep all statements clear, concise, and understandable and not crowd information and thoughts together. As worksheets are completed, the auditor must maintain a neat appearance for the papers, with special attention to clearly printing worksheet titles, headings, and names and to keeping all pages uniform in appearance and use.[6]

2. Above all, findings and data must be recorded and documented accurately.[7]

3. The auditor's innovativeness will be put to the test in designing economical usage of worksheets.[8] A good auditor will not miss an opportunity to combine on one worksheet information that may have been recorded on two or three. This consolidation also enables the auditor to comprehend the findings better and to organize data more efficiently. Properly organized worksheets help the auditor avoid collecting an endless amount of unrelated information and focus on assembling material relevant to the project's objectives.[9]

4. Worksheets must be reviewed constantly for incompleteness.[10] During the daily rush of the field work, it is easy to skip a step or fail to clarify a

finding. The auditor should review worksheets faithfully for completeness.

5. Worksheets should be organized around the audit program.[11] Each program step provides the framework for the design of a new worksheet. The auditor should describe the purpose of each discrete audit step briefly and relate it to the program so as to provide a train of thought when the working papers of each step are picked up weeks and months later.

6. A valuable procedure is to prepare a condensed summary of each audit program step as it is completed.[12] These small, concise reports provide an analysis while the auditor's mind is attuned to that step's work; help tie all the program steps together; cause a full review of the working papers for each step for completeness, accuracy, and supporting documentation, and become an extremely useful tool in the writing of the audit report.

7. All working papers, when finally assembled, should be indexed and cross-referenced.[13] Indexing may take many forms, but it should be as simple as possible. Cross-referencing leaves little room for variation either in terms of how or how rigorously it is done. Report findings must be cross-referenced with working papers and the latter cross-referenced with one another.

8. With the report completed, all materials associated with the audit must be assembled. The order of assembly may vary; however, the standard format usually involves this sequence: table of contents, audit report and summarized supporting material, audit replies, statement of scope and objectives, time budget report, and all working papers sorted either by the steps of the audit program or by sequence of use in the report.

Meeting these standards for preparing working papers will help fulfill the functions they serve in developing the audit report.

THE AUDIT REPORT

The report, as has been mentioned, is the fruit of the audit. All the hard work of the programs may be sacrificed unnecessarily on the steps of managerial neglect if the audit report fails to capture top management's attention and motivate them and department heads to implement its recommendations. For an audit report to become an attention getter and motivator, it must meet certain basic criteria.

1. The audit report must be absolutely accurate.[14,15] If the auditor does not know with certainty that a finding is true, it should be researched further or dropped. The report must be based on hard, factual evidence. The auditor seldom will be more embarrassed or internal auditing's credibility more damaged than for some aspect of the report to be proved wrong.

2. The report must be written in a clear, orderly manner with ideas, findings, and recommendations developed in a logical, straightforward, understandable format.[16,17] Readers should be provided enough background information to be able to comprehend the problem being discussed and to be able to place it into perspective with other activities and issues in the hospital and the audited department.

3. The report must be concise and focus on significant issues. To be concise, it should avoid mentioning ideas, findings, recommendations, words, and sentences that do not help develop the significant issues it is addressing. The auditor must focus on the major issues of importance to top management and avoid inserting items of less consequence that may be worked out with department heads.

4. The report must be made available to top management on a timely basis in order to provide a good motivation for action.[18] However, it must not be rushed to completion. Critically important problems requiring quick management action can be dealt with by interim, progress reports.

5. The audit report should have a professional, courteous tone that takes into consideration the feelings of the department's management and personnel. When possible, it should present a positive theme rather than appear as a negative, condemning police action. Corrective actions that department managers agreed to, and perhaps implemented, should be discussed fully in the report to demonstrate middle management's desire to accomplish departmental goals. Further, a report that tells top management many operating problems have been solved already is the type of document most hospital directors receive too seldom.

6. Last, the report must be persuasive.[19] All of the above points will assist in this, but the auditor must make every effort to sell the audit's recommendations.

The meeting of these basic criteria ensures the report will be given serious attention by the hospital's top management and the department heads. The cumulative effect of many professionally prepared reports will be to develop confidence in the internal auditing function at all levels of hospital management.

These criteria apply to the two types of reporting—oral and written—with which the internal auditor will have to deal. Oral reporting is used in many ways. It frequently is the natural outcome of working with and around people. Oral reporting often is expedient in dealing with department management. Brief visits with the manager to report the audit's progress and to discuss findings and possible solutions to problems help to maintain good rapport. Oral reports may be made where there are urgent needs for management action. The report should adhere to the criteria for reporting, for the discovery of a critical problem may not arouse management's attention if the auditor fails to prepare properly for the report. Oral reporting often is a supplement to written reports. Internal auditors often will have to explain some aspects of the report not comprehended readily. Oral reports have many uses, and internal auditors must present them effectively.

The formal written report is the ultimate reporting method for all audits.[20] Written interim and final reports provide a record for everyone in the hospital's administration to read and evaluate.[21] The impact of a well-prepared written report will evoke responses from many levels of management, starting at the department level. The report declares in writing the auditor's findings, recommendations, and opinions. This important step of documentation may take many forms. The written audit report generally will follow the format below.[22] Interim reports may borrow from the format as needed.

1. The report requires a stage-setting introduction that states briefly that an audit of a particular department has been completed, with the date. The department's size and activities and the audit's major conclusions should be summarized.
2. The purpose of the audit must be explained. A general statement can be made followed by a listing of the objectives, which should have been provided in writing as a part of the auditor's instructions.
3. The scope of the audit should be stated. The auditor should specify what areas and activities were covered and point out those omitted that might bear on top management's use of the report.
4. The auditor should express an opinion as to how well the department has been operating. A manager performing a similar review certainly would form an opinion and the auditor, acting in top management's place, should provide the administration with an overall assessment for consideration. The auditor must be prepared, however, to support the opinion with accurate findings.
5. The reader of the report now is prepared for the more detailed findings. The auditor's opinion should have aroused the reader's curiosity as to the findings that led to such a result. The audit's findings must support all opinions and recommendations and must not cover unrelated points and minutiae. The findings must be edited carefully to cover all points of importance to top management and leave out less important findings and recommendations that should be worked out with the department manager. The auditor may choose to emphasize findings that are a positive reflection on the department as well as those that are negative. This is a debatable point. Inclusion of positive findings tends to produce a pseudoobjectivity and balance that may be soothing when the negative points are considered. Most audits will find that improvement is possible, thereby always having something negative to report. The only recommendation provided here is not to flatter those audited, either to influence them or to prepare them for

a doomsday report. A department that is average should be reported as such and one with an outstanding performance should be so reported. Laudatory appraisals should not become a routine part of reports unless fully merited.

All findings should be cross-referenced with working papers on the auditor's copy of the report. A question that is answered quickly and completely will attract top management's attention and increase the auditor's credibility. Many an auditor has been demoralized by pinpoint questions whose answers are buried in the worksheets. In preparing the report, the auditor must have so organized and cross-referenced all supporting workpapers and documents as to be completely confident that any question can be answered readily.

For example, during an oral presentation of a report, the auditor may criticize the handling of the purchase of certain supplies. This criticism may be supported by specifics on the many times the supply inventory has been exhausted and on the crisis situations that have resulted. A hospital director may inquire as to the causes. The auditor responds that the problem stems from ordering small quantities with irregular frequency. The hospital director inquires as to quantities and frequencies. The auditor produces a worksheet that provides an analysis of those factors. The director asks what data were used to compile the analysis. The auditor then produces detailed supporting documents such as order form copies or a computer printout. Hospital directors tend to ask many embarrassing questions if the auditor is unprepared. Be prepared.

The actual writing of audit reports must meet many established criteria. These criteria will not be covered here in favor of stressing a few key issues. It is prudent to ask another auditor to read the report before the director of internal auditing does. The more criticism, questions, and points of view that can be surfaced during the writing, the better the result will be and the better the auditor will be prepared to handle criticism and questions. Preliminary discussions should be held with the department's management on all parts of the report.[23]

The auditor may sell many of the recommendations at this point and, if unsuccessful, at least will know what counterpoints and arguments will be presented. The final report must be proofread thoroughly. The impact of a report and oral presentation can be lost quickly when it is pointed out that a column of numbers does not add up or certain figures are missing. The report distribution list agreed to during the discussion of instructions with the director of internal auditing should be reviewed carefully. Last, it is recommended that the report be sent to all involved parties and that an exit or closing conference be arranged to allow the auditor to present the material orally and respond to comments and questions.[24] Copies should be sent out early enough to allow top management and department heads to prepare but not so early that the report will have become old news before the conference.

AUDIT REPORT RESPONSE AND FOLLOW-UP

Once the audit report has been presented to the governing board or audit committee, the hospital director, and the department management, a written response should be prepared by the department head and the administrator responsible for the department. The response should detail what actions will be taken to correct problems uncovered by the audit and, in particular, should discuss all report recommendations. The response should be prepared within two to four weeks and addressed to the highest level to which the audit report was routed. The nature and tone of the response will provide the auditor with a good indication of how successful the various steps of the audit program were. A defensive, combative response that denies the problems and rejects all recommendations must be viewed as at least partly the auditor's failure to gain the confidence of the department management.[25] Reactions such as this produce a bitter struggle for top management support, with everyone losing in the end.

Regardless of how poor the department is or how outstanding the recommendations are, the governing board and/or the hospital director will not be excited about mediating between the internal auditing function and the department audited. The auditor must learn to expect some defensiveness by those audited because of their pride; however, extremely negative responses should be expected only infrequently. The auditor's role in the response phase is to monitor the time in which the reply should be made. Once a response is received the auditor must bring unsatisfactory answers to the attention of the hospital director, and perhaps the board, for decision. The auditor may present arguments supporting the points rejected by the department, but the ultimate decision lies with top management. A choice of action not recommended by the auditor can occur frequently, but the auditor must continue to supply proposals for consideration and not become fearful of rejection of some ideas.

Once all aspects of the response are agreed to, the auditor must plan a short visit to the department in the future.

Follow-up reviews are an important standard practice that essentially closes the feedback loop.[26] The auditor must allow sufficient time for the department to implement the changes. The review should be timed to permit short spot checks on performance, if needed. To do this, the changes should have been operative long enough to have built up new patterns of performance. The auditor is interested in verifying whether the agreed-to changes have been made and that they have solved the problems. Such a result is gratifying to the auditor and to top management.

With the follow-up review completed and a brief file report prepared and added to the workpapers, the director of internal auditing should evaluate the audit and auditor. Evaluation will be dealt with in detail in Chapter 17; however, it is worth noting that the internal auditing function must contribute effectively to meeting hospital and departmental goals or face possible elimination as an unnecessary burden on the institution's resources.

A WORD ON AUDIT COMMITTEES

Before moving on to Part IV and practical applications for the function, a new aspect of both internal and external auditing should be mentioned briefly. The use of formal audit committees is on the rise and has received strong support from certified public accountants and institutions such as the Securities and Exchange Commission and the New York Stock Exchange.[27]

The audit committee should be appointed by the governing body and consist of three to five board members. Audit committee members should have backgrounds that provide a broad perspective of hospital operations rather than a high degree of technical competence in accounting and finance.[28] Typical audit committee duties are:

1. to meet with the external auditor to review the annual audit and management letter, the scope of audit engagements, annual financial statements, hospital management control systems, and the staffing of accounting and financial areas, including internal auditing[29,30]
2. to meet with the director of internal auditing to review that office's reports and the adequacy of its program and staffing
3. to meet with the hospital's financial and administrative officers to review implementing recommendations made by the external and internal auditors
4. to approve the selection of the external auditor and the director of internal auditing

An audit committee, to be effective, should meet a number of times a year to cover specific topics selected from the duties cited above. The committee requires the support of the board and the hospital's administration to achieve its best results. It should have a broad scope for its reviews so it can evaluate all the hospital. It should study carefully the adequacy of the external and internal auditing reports and the performance of the hospital's administration. The audit committee provides board level attention to all matters that come under its review, thereby providing the governing body with greatly improved information and supervisory capabilities. The committee's end product is the improved quality and quantity of communications with the board, the external and internal auditors, and the hospital's administration.

CONCLUSION

Reporting audit findings in a manner that is communicative and motivating is not easy. Hospital administrators must be sold on the idea of taking action to solve problems surfaced by audits. Top management must be receptive to audit reports and be prepared to support their findings and recommendations. Both the auditor and the administration have important responsibilities for making the reporting experience successful.

SUMMARY OF PART III

Chapter 9 concludes the introduction of hospital internal auditing theory and practice. The hospital that adopts these concepts will have laid a secure foundation for the development of an effective internal auditing capability. Parts IV and V will concentrate on the equally important practical applications of internal auditing in hospitals and teaching medical centers. Administrators are encouraged to ask themselves if their hospitals can meet the tests internal auditors will apply. Numerous thought-provoking internal audit checklists are provided that should simplify the task. Internal auditors will find the practical applications and checklists are good starting points for examining current audit programs for improvement and for designing new ones.

NOTES

1. Lawrence B. Sawyer, *The Practice of Modern Internal Auditing* (Orlando, Fla.: The Institute of Internal Auditors, Inc., 1973), pp. 330–331.

2. Victor Z. Brink, James A. Cashin, and Herbert Witt, *Modern Internal Auditing: An Operational Approach* (New York: The Ronald Press Company, 1973), p. 620.

3. Sawyer, op. cit., p. 332.

4. Ibid., p. 331.

5. Brink, op. cit., pp. 620–621.

6. Comptroller General of the United States, *Standards for Audit of Governmental Organizations, Programs, Activities, and Functions* (Washington, D.C.: General Accounting Office, 1972), p. 37.

7. Brink, op. cit., p. 622.

8. Sawyer, op. cit., p. 334.

9. Brink, op. cit., p. 622.

10. Comptroller of the U.S., op. cit., p. 37.

11. Sawyer, op. cit., pp. 335–336.

12. Ibid., p. 339.

13. Ibid., pp. 340–341.

14. Brink, op. cit., p. 632

15. Sawyer, op. cit., pp. 358–359.

16. Ibid., pp. 359–362.

17. E. N. Carlson, "The S.R.O.F. System of Report Writing," *Internal Auditor*, December 1975, pp. 19–26.

18. Comptroller of the U.S., op. cit., p. 41.

19. R. F. Fitzgerald, "Influential Reports: Technical Skills, Not Personal Style," *Internal Auditor*, October 1973, pp. 44–45.

20. A. E. Marien, "The Internal Control Function, Part IV: The Internal Auditor Reports," *Hospital Financial Management*, June 1971, p. 12.

21. Comptroller of the U.S., op. cit., p. 39.

22. Sawyer, op. cit., pp. 364–372.

23. J. A. C. Higgins, "The Effective Audit Report—Our Most Important Product," *Internal Auditor*, June 1973, pp. 48–49.

24. D. S. Rogers, "The Audit Report—Ambassador of Internal Auditing," *Internal Auditor*, August 1977, pp. 34–35.

25. F. E. Mints, "Cooperative Auditing—The Key to the Future," *Internal Auditor*, December 1973, pp. 32–44.

26. A. J. Hallinan, "There Is No Escape From Follow-Up Except . . . ," *Internal Auditor*, February 1974, pp. 31–38.

27. R. L. Colegrove, "The Functions and Responsibilities of the Corporate Audit Committee," *Internal Auditor*, June 1976, p. 16.

28. N. E. Auerbach, "Audit Committees—New Corporate Institution," *Financial Executive*, September 1973, p. 96.

29. N. E. Auerbach, "ABCs of Audit Committees," *Financial Executive*, October 1976, p. 24.

30. S. D. Harlan, Jr., "How to Make the Audit Committee Work Best for All Concerned," *World*, Spring 1974, p. 22.

A Guide for the Practical Application of Internal Auditing in Hospitals

Chapter 10

Evaluating Top Management Performance

Part IV marks the departure from theory and practice and a turn to practical applications of management, operations, compliance, and financial internal auditing in hospitals. These types of internal auditing are applied to many of the wide range of hospital activities and operations. It is not possible to include all applications, but internal auditors and hospital administrators are encouraged to seek out other uses for the function. Many of the applications in Part IV can serve as a basis for these innovations because the auditing methods and checkpoints provided can be used in most hospital departments.

PRACTICAL ASPECTS OF INTERNAL AUDITING

Internal auditing has many practical applications in hospitals and most of them share common checkpoints. A checkpoint is a specific matter of interest regarding a particular subject that internal auditors should review during an audit. Since internal audit programs appraise elements that exist in most departments and functions, such as written procedures or physical facilities, auditors are obliged to review the same checkpoints again and again. A listing of the more frequent audit checkpoints used in hospital departments appears below. These common checkpoints are presented here to minimize the number of times they will need to be mentioned during discussions of specific topics in Parts IV and V. These points always should be referred to during the preparation of audit programs. A number of the discussions of practical applications that follow will include some of these checkpoints both to keep them visible and to demonstrate their usage.

Organization and Internal Control

1. Who does the administrator of the department report to? Is this the right person to report to? How often are reports made and in what form? Are they clear, accurate, representative, and timely?

2. How is the department organized? Is there an organizational chart? Does it provide for good internal controls? Are areas of authority and responsibility indicated clearly? Is it centralized or decentralized and to what advantage?
3. How is the department's work coordinated with the rest of the hospital? Are the interdepartmental organizational relationships clear and satisfactory?
4. What internal controls are used? Where needed, do they accomplish their purpose economically?
5. What records are generated by the department? Do they promote efficient work accomplishment?

Policies and Procedures

1. Are all departmental policies and procedures committed to writing? Who prepared them and were they approved by the governing board? Are they followed?
2. Are the policies and procedures kept complete and current? Are they adequate? Do they deal effectively with patient care needs?
3. Are departmental policies and procedures in harmony with those of the hospital?
4. Are there too many or too few policies and procedures? Are there procedures for handling all routine work decisions? How are nonroutine decisions made?
5. Have all policies and procedures been communicated clearly to employees and patients? Are they aware of the policies and procedures?

Goals, Objectives, and Planning

1. Have clear goals and objectives been established for the department? Are they in writing?
2. Are the goals and objectives measurable and achievable? Are they in harmony with those of the hospital?
3. Are departmental plans committed to writing? Is there sufficient planning and how is it integrated with the overall planning process of the hospital?

Staffing

1. Are employee interviewing and screening procedures adequate?
2. Are employees properly certified?
3. What provisions are made for daily supervision and training?
4. Are employees routinely moved about when there is not enough work available to keep everyone fully employed?

5. Are there adequate job descriptions? Are there adequate productivity measures?
6. How good is employee morale? What is the employee turnover rate? How are breaks and absences handled and with what impact on internal control?
7. Is the area staffed properly with adequate numbers of employees who are qualified and capable of performing at expected levels?

Facilities

1. Does the department's location contribute to accomplishing its goals?
2. Is the department adequately equipped? Is the equipment modern and in good operating order?
3. Does the department have good communication systems? In particular, are there effective uses of telephone communication capabilities?
4. Is there enough space for employees and patients? Does the area and arrangement of space promote efficiency?
5. Is the environment of the area safe and does it promote efficiency? Is it clean, well lighted, and temperature controlled?
6. What security measures exist to safeguard the space, equipment, employees, and patients from crime?

IN SUPPORT OF MANAGEMENT AUDITING

The idea of internal auditors evaluating hospital administrators is new and controversial. The hospital's entire condition is dependent on its administrators doing a good job of managing. The best efforts of department managers, physicians, and internal auditors will be thwarted if top management fails to plan, organize, staff, direct, and control hospital affairs effectively. It is for this reason that internal auditing must evaluate hospital administrators. The internal auditing function must provide the governing board complete and accurate information on the institution's progress toward achieving its goals—goals that can be achieved only by superior administrative leadership. Hospital administrators must learn to rely on internal auditors for timely, professional, and insightful appraisals of their management leadership performance. Expensive outside consultants often are paid to provide constructive criticism of this nature after hospitals encounter significant management operating difficulties. Internal auditors can provide similar services at lower costs and avoid the development of severe operating problems.

Internal auditors must be prepared to evaluate management. To be able to perform an audit of this nature, they must achieve a high level of knowledge of hospital administration. This will require them to have studied hospital management and preferably actually to have participated at some time in such administration. Management auditing is a new field for internal auditing and exacting guidelines have not been developed to help the auditor. Some experts argue that auditing management is too broad an undertaking and that it is too difficult to measure effectively.[1,2] These difficulties also are challenges that the internal auditing profession can rise to meet. Auditing management performance must be regarded as the ultimate challenge for hospital administrators to accept and for internal auditors to provide. Without this level of evaluation, hospitals cannot expect to receive the maximum benefit the function can provide.

A NOTE ON MANAGEMENT LEADERSHIP

Before continuing with a more detailed development of auditing management, the critical importance of the administration's leadership role must be examined. Management literature has much to say about leadership but frequently neglects the issue of excellence versus mediocrity. The public and its elected representatives have found the health care industry run in an unacceptable manner. It may be conjectured that many of the industry's problems are the result of widespread mediocre management. This must be close to the case and for this reason mediocrity has a great impact on the internal auditing function. Internal auditing will find it tough going in hospitals where mediocrity best describes management's leadership role.

Internal auditing is a positive force, seeking out and supporting improvement in all phases of hospital operations. If the function seeks excellence both in the professional performance of its work and, at the same time, in hospital operation, administrations that do not identify with the pursuit of such a goal will block and frustrate the efforts of internal auditors. The significance of excellence versus mediocrity need not be elaborated further. Where internal auditors find mediocrity, they must make every effort to encourage a change in management philosophy and perspective.

MANAGEMENT AUDITING

Management auditing requires analysis of top management's performance in planning, organizing, staffing, directing, and controlling.

Planning

Planning is a relatively new concept in management. Formal short, intermediate, and long-range planning was recognized as an important management function less than 100 years ago when the size and complexity of enterprises began to grow rapidly. As yet, planning has no generally accepted meaning.[3] For present purposes, the American Management Association's definition of planning is suitable: Planning is a commitment to action on an orderly, realistic, systematic basis; it is a reasoned choice of courses of action.[4] Planning is concerned with the future. It is a process that should be continuous and must be structured to provide consistency among individual plans. Hospitals can benefit from sound management planning and should not be without it.

The internal auditor should examine top management's plans and planning process to verify how adequately this vital function has been fulfilled.[5] The internal auditor must watch for pitfalls in planning. Some examples of common deficiencies and limitations are:

1. There may be a lack of genuine top management support and interest in planning. Hospital administrators often may avoid the level of involvement required for good planning, with the consequence that the quality of the activity diminishes. Delegating the process leads to inferior plans.
2. Planning may be done by a centralized, top-down process. Plans thus generated often are prepared for top management's approval, rather than with the hospital's operations, in mind. Such planning seldom reflects realistic assessments of the needs and capabilities of departments and personnel.
3. Planning may be based on poorly prepared forecasts—the basic premises upon which it proceeds. Equally important, management information used in planning may be inaccurate, misleading, or missing.
4. Plans may be consistently conservative, with the result that opportunities seldom are exploited fully and, as a consequence, hospitals are not pressed toward their best performance.
5. Planning may be deficient in assessing critically the various avenues for change and fail to provide adequate detail for establishing means for controlling progress toward objectives and goals.
6. The planning process may be overly zealous, with the result that its costs are unjustifiably high. Excessive amounts of time and money may be poured into planning not only at the hospital's major levels but also descending to the depths of its organization. Hospital administrators may be expected to routinely commit 25 to 30 percent of their time to planning.[6]
7. The planning process may become a traditional function that does not build on past accomplishments and press on to new achievements.
8. Plans may become restrictive and inflexible. Management at all levels may be robbed of initiative and the development of innovative ideas may be stifled.
9. Plans, goals, objectives, and standards may be communicated poorly throughout the hospital with the result that no one knows what is going on.

The internal auditor may discover any of these deficiencies and limitations during the review of top management's planning process.

A second internal auditing perspective is to assess the apparent worth of top management's plans. A number of internal auditing benchmarks are available:

1. Top management plans should provide for positive change in the hospital's operations. Goals, objectives, and standards must be realistic and be set high enough to produce motivation.
2. Plans must result in improved operations. Improvement may be evaluated by using literature available on hospital management. The purpose of proposed plans must be stated clearly in order to assess their worthiness. The steps to be followed in fulfilling the planned goals and objectives must be documented.
3. It must be apparent that all plans are coordinated with each other and that the result enhances the hospital's operations.
4. Resources assigned to each plan should be reasonable and sufficient.
5. Top management should have an established track record of coping successfully with problems as they arise. All too often management may do a good job of planning only to become unresponsive to problems that develop as the reality of day-to-day operations is confronted.

Internal auditors can evaluate top management's planning performance in terms of both process and actual plans generated. The factors cited above are starting places for internal auditors to develop their own methods and checkpoints. This can be done only if auditors properly prepare themselves by studying planning in general and hospital planning in particular.

Organizing

Organizing hospital functions, resources, and personnel is a challenging management responsibility.[7] The importance of the organizing role has grown along the same pattern as that of planning.[8] The rising number of administrators in hospitals is believed to be the direct result of the increased complexity of the institutions' organization and less closely related to their overall size.[9] If these findings are true, top management's ability to deal successfully with the complexities of modern hospitals can have a direct influence on the need for increased resource allocations for more administrators. Hospital administrators should be expected to spend about 5 percent of their time on organization matters.[10]

The requirement for organization grows out of the human need for cooperation and coordination. Because hospitals are so complex, effective organization is even more essential. A hospital's organizational setting includes the formal and informal structure of roles and relationships of its employees. The organizational process

> embraces a multitude of activities that result in the establishment of authority-responsibility relationships and the interrelating of human and other resources in such a way that the work performed will lead to the fulfillment of the organization's objectives. The activities include the establishment of authority and responsibility relationships, the division of work, the delegation of that work, and the coordination of work effort.[11]

Hospitals must be organized properly to achieve maximum effectiveness and efficiency in all operating components.

The role of internal auditing in evaluating top management's organizational setting has just begun to develop.[12] Internal audit checkpoints have not been published to an extent that can be drawn on here for possible application in hospitals. However, it is possible to propose checkpoints based on a review of literature on hospital organization:[13]

1. Top management should have documented the hospital's structure by creating formal organization charts of line responsibilities and staff functions. The charts should be examined for currency and completeness. The exact relationship between positions and functions on the charts should be documented in writing, with attention directed to delegated authority and responsibility.[14] Written job descriptions should support the intended organizational relationships. Spans of control should be examined for undue breadth.[15]
2. The auditor should acquire a working knowledge of top management's organizing techniques in dealing with the medical, paramedical, nursing, and support staffs. This knowledge can be acquired from interviews and deduced from operating manuals. Findings should be presented to the hospital's director to be certain they fairly represent top management's intentions.[16]
3. The hospital's organization should complement and support: (a) hospital goals and objectives; (b) top management's leadership style; (c) all operating levels of the hospital, tying them together both horizontally and vertically in a common bond toward achieving goals and objectives; and (d) employee good will and foster staff identification with and integration of the institution's goals and objectives.[17]
4. The governing board, the administration, the medical staff, and the hospital's staff should be examined to determine their roles in the organizing process.[18]

5. Specific signs of sound organization are: the ability to adapt to change, the ability to attract and retain good management talent, the presence of good employee morale and motivation, the absence of internal conflict, a minimum of duplication of resources, an apparent economical operation, and a continuing process that reviews the existing organization for needed change.
6. Specific signs of poor organization are: frequent plan changes, a lack of arranged job succession, late decisions, inadequate information, poor accountability, excessive meetings and communications, a tolerance of incompetence, wage and salary inequities, and purposeless redundancy.[19]

The internal auditor will have to piece together information from many sources to document an evaluation of the hospital's organization. The auditor always should review findings with the hospital director. Instances of conflict between what the director believes to be the case and what is found during the information gathering process must be resolved before any evaluation can be made. Actual evaluation must rely on the internal auditor's education and background on organization. The auditor can draw on a great deal of literature on organization in general and hospital organization in particular.

In the end, the auditor may conclude that the hospital's organizing philosophies and techniques have not been stated clearly, that the organization may be poorly documented, that it does not glue the institution together into an effective and efficient unit of operation, that it has produced operating problems, and that the roles of the administration and staff are not defined clearly. Findings such as these occur all too often.

Auditing management's performance in organizing the hospital is a challenging task, but one that can lead to many improvements in fine tuning specific organizing methods and techniques. Top management should welcome an objective evaluation of performance, and internal auditors must prepare themselves to produce professional evaluations.

Staffing

With the problems of organization resolved, the next questions are: who will be given the various organization responsibilities, what kind of people will be needed, how many, where will they be found, and how will they be trained, supervised, and compensated?[20]

The growing size and complexity of modern hospitals has increased the importance of proper staffing significantly. The health care industry is dependent on acquiring adequate numbers of skilled personnel.[21] Hospital directors and governing boards are responsible for establishing suitable personnel policies, for selecting the administrative staff and for ensuring that the institution has an effectively functioning personnel department. Staffing and personnel management have been the focus of much attention. Internal auditors will find it easy to acquire a good background on the subject before starting the project because of the abundance of helpful literature. In general, an audit of top management's performance of staffing should cover at least three broad areas:[22]

1. The internal auditor should document hospital personnel policies developed by top management. They should be in writing, complete, and up to date, and provide a basis for good personnel selection and management. The policies should result in many written procedures that specifically cover the next two points.
2. The internal auditor should review recruiting policies and procedures and the actual performance of processes for obtaining adequate numbers of qualified personnel on an economical and timely basis. In particular, the auditor will want to evaluate top management's staffing process, its resourcefulness and success at tapping both internal and external sources of personnel recruiting, and whether it provides for proper and adequate uses of job analysis techniques that generate position descriptions and specifications. The auditor also must determine whether recruiting is in compliance with employment laws, whether actual selection methods make good use of background information acquired from the applications, interviewing, and testing and, last, whether there are new employee orientation procedures.
3. The internal auditor should evaluate programs for improving employee performance and retention. The auditor should appraise employee evaluation methods and training and development programs. Wage and salary administration should be studied carefully since much of the hospital's cost of operation involves payroll. The auditor also should review programs on employee health, safety, retirement, and fringe benefits.

Internal auditing can make a contribution to improving hospital staffing policies and procedures. The auditor may find the administration has not directed enough attention to those elements and that its efforts in hiring and employee retention are costly and ineffective. Everyone concerned with the hospital's performance should welcome a review of staffing.

Directing

With the hospital's plans prepared and its organization developed and staffed, the point of getting the work done emerges. Directing has assumed a new importance in modern hospitals, taking an estimated 25 percent of administrative time.[23] Outdated management leadership techniques that were mechanical and autocratic have been replaced by theories of motivation, leadership, and communication. While there is much literature on organizational behavior, leadership, motivation, and communication, few findings or theories are agreed on. The internal auditor should be familiar with texts on organizational behavior in general and on hospital leadership, motivation, and communication in particular. The auditor will have to rely on these readings, practical experience, and good judgment to be able to evaluate top management's directing performance at all levels.

Supporting documentation will be difficult to acquire. The auditor may be able to make use of an employee attitude survey to uncover staff perceptions of top management's leadership and supervisory styles, worker discontent and lack of motivation, absence of cohesiveness and a sense of belonging to and contributing to the hospital's performance, and problems in communication. Problems the auditor believes to exist, and that may be supported by objective evidence, should be discussed with the hospital's administration in a workshop atmosphere.

Top management must be encouraged to evaluate its styles and methods of direction objectively and make decisions on their suitability or need for change. An audit checklist cannot be provided. Directing activities vary broadly among hospital administrators. Most research and model building in this area is in its infancy and provides no agreed-on methods that can be expected to produce similar results in different circumstances. Even though directing is a difficult area to audit, hospitals cannot help but be benefited by efforts to appraise it. Both top management and the auditor may be surprised at the results of attitude surveys and general discussions of issues that compose the directing activity.

Controlling

While the previous four management functions clearly are interrelated, management control provides the framework for tying them together. Top management is responsible for monitoring hospital operations, comparing results with planned goals, and determining what further courses of action are needed. Internal auditors traditionally have been concerned with internal control and should be well prepared to evaluate management efforts. Good management control of resource inputs, activities, and outputs is crucial to ensuring that patients receive the best of care at reasonable costs. Research indicates hospital administrators invest 10 percent of their time on control matters.[24]

The nature of control is important. Too often "control" conveys the idea of holding back or restraining, keeping employees on the right track. While this is an appropriate interpretation, it places undue emphasis on control's negative, inhibiting characteristics. A more effective perspective views control as a guiding and motivating force that propels employees forward toward specific goals, not restraining them.[25] Good control, rather than keeping things from happening, actually has as its purpose making them happen.[26]

The control process should be documented by top management. Internal auditors should find that the administration has completed a number of steps in gaining control:

1. Hospital directors must establish performance standards clearly and in measurable terms. Employees must know what is expected of them to be able to determine how well they are performing. Criteria set by top managers also reveal their personal standards, which the auditor must try to evaluate as to their suitability in the health care environment.

2. The internal auditor must be certain that the performance standards have been communicated effectively throughout the hospital. Clear communication always has proved to be a difficult task. The auditor should interview employees, or survey a sample of the staff, as to their understanding of the standards.

3. Once employees know what is expected of them, the administration must provide for the collection of data on performance and arrange for its processing into management reports.[27] The value of usable information cannot be understated. It is the one step in the control cycle that cannot be controlled absolutely by top management. Hospital directors set and communicate standards, compare reported performance with the standards, and decide on and implement corrective action, but they are not involved directly in data gathering and its processing into reports. Hospital directors may plan the systems for data gathering and processing, but in the end they are dependent on employees and systems and procedures to handle the management information process properly. Internal auditors can play an important role in validating management information.

4. Once good information is in the hands of management, the results should be compared to planned goals and standards. Deviations from plans must be noted and examined for the need of further action. Deviations may occur in either direction; i.e., performance may be found to be much better or much worse than planned. Both types of deviation must be analyzed.

5. Once deviations are found and analyzed, a correcting course of action must be set. Top management must choose the type of action and its direction, timing, and place as well as identify and commit resources to implementing it. Internal auditors must assure themselves that top management explored alternate solutions and, after selecting a course of action, committed themselves to carrying it out in a proper and timely fashion.

6. The need for correction and the course of action selected must be communicated to those concerned. Corrective action often is a sensitive matter. Personnel may have to be disciplined or even discharged. At the very least,

corrective action often implies failure except where performance has been better than planned. Top management must make an effort to retain employees' good will during the correction process. To do this, the positive side of the action must be presented. Internal auditors should review the nature of corrective actions and try to determine whether they did improve operations and were implemented without undue disruption of employee work and morale. These last two checkpoints can be evaluated by examining productivity during the implementation period and interviewing employees as to their perception of the corrective action.

Effective management control cannot be achieved without meeting the criteria of the above six steps. As mentioned in step 3, hospital directors often are very dependent on the reports they receive for controlling. If the reports are untimely, inaccurate, incomplete, or even falsified, management loses control. Internal auditors can play a valuable role in validating the accuracy, representativeness, and usefulness of management information.

VALIDATING MANAGEMENT INFORMATION

Reporting systems can encounter a number of problems for which internal auditors should be on the alert:[28]

1. Reports to management may be too complex and contain far too much data and too little information. Reporting formats may be unnecessarily complicated and difficult to analyze. Internal auditors should evaluate reports for clarity and conciseness.
2. Top management may receive reports with information that is of no use. This is a common problem where reports are sent routinely to everyone. Few of those who receive them will bother to review them. Internal auditors should review report distributions for applicability. Frequently, hospitals can realize a considerable benefit by cutting back on the number of copies of reports and thereby save paper, printing costs, and handling time.
3. Reports may place much emphasis on quantitative matters such as dollars and provide no information as to why or what caused the numbers to be what they are. Top management needs to know not only the quantities but also the underlying conditions. Internal auditors should review the processes by which the reports are assembled and recommend to the preparers that they provide explanations for the figures.
4. Reports might include too little information, contain incorrect data, or have summaries that conceal poor performance or flatter a department. Hospital directors may not be aware they are not informed of everything. Omissions

are common and difficult to detect. Reports containing wrong or misleading information are equally hard to detect. Internal auditors should review all phases of data gathering and its assembly to assure top management the reports can be believed.

5. Reporting requirements may be unclear. Personnel must know to whom, what, and how often to report. Auditors should analyze the entire reporting structure to be certain top management is informed of all phases of the hospital's operations.
6. Hospitals should use modern methods for generating reports. In particular, internal auditors should be alert for applications of electronic data processing. Even small hospitals can lease or share computing capabilities that improve accuracy of data collections and the overall quality of the reports

Internal auditors will discover many more audit checkpoints for the management information system. The above six cover many of the more common problems and form a basis for many other findings once the audit is begun.

Internal auditors should be prepared to evaluate top management's control of hospitals. The significance of effective control is clear and the interdependence of all management functions is apparent. Control cannot exist without planning, organizing, staffing, and directing.

CONCLUSION

Management auditing is a new activity that has not been accepted fully by internal auditors or hospital administrators. Traditionally, internal auditing reported *to* management, not *on* management. The need for professionally performed internal audits of management is clear. Hospitals frequently employ consultants to evaluate management at considerable expense. They should develop the same capability internally in the form of management auditing. Public accounting firms frequently provide opinions on administrators' performance in the form of management information letters. If offering these types of opinions is a commonly accepted practice for public accountants, why not add it as an internal auditing function as well? Management auditing is supported by the new *Standards for the Professional Practice of Internal Auditing.* The standards clearly state that internal auditors have as a responsibility the well-being of the hospital, not merely reporting to management. Internal auditors must learn to evaluate management for the good of the institution.

NOTES

1. C. H. Smith, R. A. Lanier, and M. E. Taylor, "The Need for and Scope of the Audit of Management: A Survey of Attitudes," *Accounting Review,* April 1972, pp. 270–283.

2. E. H. Morse, Jr., "Comments on the Survey of Attitudes on Management Auditing," *Accounting Review,* January 1973, pp. 120–125.

3. George A. Steiner, *Top Management Planning* (New York: The Macmillan Company, 1969), p. 5.

4. Roy A. Lindberg and Theodore Cohn, *Operations Auditing* (New York: American Management Association, 1972), p. 56.

5. S. D. Watson, "Internal Auditing Viewed from the Top," *Internal Auditor,* December 1973, p. 27.

6. Rockwell Schulz and Alton C. Johnson, *Management of Hospitals* (New York: McGraw-Hill Book Company, 1976), p. 131.

7. Jonathon S. Rakich, Beaufort B. Lonest, Jr., and Thomas R. O'Donovan, *Managing Health Care Organizations* (Philadelphia: W. B. Saunders Company, 1977), p. 189.

8. Lindberg, op. cit., p. 77.

9. Wolf Heydebrand, *Hospital Bureaucracy: A Comparative Study of Organizations* (New York: Dunellen Publishing Company, 1973), p. 393.

10. Schulz, op. cit., p. 131.

11. Rakich, op. cit., p. 139.

12. Lindberg, op. cit., p. 79.

13. The Institute of Internal Auditors, "The Internal Auditor's Review of Organizational Control," *Research Committee Report 18,* Institute of Internal Auditors, Inc., p. 12.

14. G. McIntyre, "Auditing for Management Control," *Internal Auditor,* June 1975, p. 38.

15. Lindberg, op. cit., p. 81.

16. Ralph Rowbotton et al., *Hospital Organizations* (London: Heinemann Educational Books, Ltd., 1973), pp. 73–171.

17. Victor Z. Brink, James A. Cashin, and Herbert Witt, *Modern Internal Auditing: An Operational Approach* (New York: The Ronald Press Company, 1973), p. 50.

18. Rakich, op. cit., pp. 186–194.

19. Lindberg, op. cit., p. 79.

20. Brink, op. cit., pp. 50–51.

21. Rakich, op. cit., p. 203.

22. Ibid., pp. 203–231.

23. Schulz, op. cit., p. 131.

24. Ibid., p. 131.

25. Addison C. Bennett, ed., *Improving the Effectiveness of Hospital Management* (New York: Preston Anglearn Publishing Company, 1972), p. 105.

26. J. G. Morfin, "The Function of Control and Internal Control," *Internal Auditor,* February 1973, p. 42.

27. McIntyre, op. cit., p. 41.

28. Bennett, op. cit., pp. 112–116.

Chapter 11

Operations Auditing of Patient Care Areas

It is apparent the results of the management audit will influence the topics of the remaining chapters of Part IV. The reader must be aware continually there is no substitute for sound administration in hospitals. This chapter presents practical applications of operations auditing methods for the patient care area. Patient care is the entire focus for hospitals, and their efforts to perform that function well must be reviewed thoroughly by internal auditors. The governing board and administration must be informed of how well (or poorly) all the operating components of the hospital provide the care.

The starting place for an operations audit is the review of operating manuals and supplementary written instructions for the department to be audited. These written systems and procedures must be examined for accuracy, completeness, and operating soundness. After a preliminary evaluation of the procedures, the internal auditor determines the levels of employee compliance with the written procedures and appraises the inadequacy in fulfilling the hospital's mission of patient care.

AUDITING ADMITTING AND DISCHARGE PROCEDURES

The most important ingredients of any hospital system or procedure are the patients and their care. All findings must be evaluated with this goal in mind. Any soundly conceived business system that in the end does not take the care of patient and family into consideration fails this test and must be brought to the attention of top administration for correction.

Admitting and Discharge Policies

Internal auditors must evaluate the adequacy of written policies for admitting and discharging patients, how they were generated, who is responsible for keeping them up to date, the method used, and whether employees are aware of them. Following are starting points for auditors to design custom tailored audits for their hospitals.

General

1. Are there any particular types of illnesses that will be not admitted?
2. What is the policy for emergency admissions? What priority do they have over other admissions and how is the procedure protected from abuses of the privilege?
3. What liability release forms are required?
4. What patient classification system exists and does it describe the various patient groups adequately?
5. Are patients routinely segregated by type of admitting diagnosis?

Financial

1. What policy is used to admit charity patients and how does the hospital control its charity load?
2. What is the policy on requiring advance deposits from patients without third-party payor coverage?
3. What is the screening process for determining patient ability to pay, for acquiring financial information, and for verifying insurance coverage?
4. How are patients handled for readmission when they have outstanding balances?
5. What is the policy for discounts on hospital bills?

Organization of Admissions

1. Is the admitting office located in one area under one supervisor or decentralized to other buildings and areas under several supervisors? Is the form of organization effective?
2. To whom do the supervisors of admissions report?
3. What authority and responsibilities do the supervisors have?
4. Is the organizational pattern documented and do all employees know and understand it?
5. What provision is there for coordinating other hospital operations with admissions?

Staffing Admissions

1. Do adequate job descriptions exist for all employee positions and do they complement the existing organization? Do employees know their jobs?

2. What provision is there for monitoring employee turnover, absenteeism, and overtime? How are staff shortages dealt with? Are temporary employees used or do persons from other departments fill in temporarily in admissions?
3. What provisions exist for orientation of new employees, training, performance evaluation, wage and salary administration, and staff benefits?
4. Do employees appear motivated, do they identify with the hospital's goals, and are they loyal?
5. What provisions exist for employee feedback?

Physical Facilities for Admissions

1. Where is the admissions office located in relation to the lobby, main entrances, emergency room, medical records, the business and cashier offices, and patient and physician traffic patterns?
2. Is there sufficient space to provide for patient privacy during interviews and has adequate space been assigned for waiting areas, toilets, equipment, records storage, and personnel?
3. Are operating conditions safe and comfortable and do they encourage good employee performance? Is the area clean, climate controlled, nicely decorated and furnished, and well lighted, and are there enough clearly marked exits and sufficient aisle space?
4. Is admissions equipped properly with business machines, copy machines, and telephones?
5. Is the area laid out to facilitate a normal flow of operation?

Admitting Procedures

1. Is there a system of preregistering elective admission patients and, if so, do the forms and instructions sent to patients provide enough information for the hospital and the individuals?
2. Is the current census known at all times and are available beds well controlled?
3. Do admitting forms provide complete information for all hospital business systems? What is the distribution of the forms?
4. How are patient clothes and valuables handled? How are advance payments handled?
5. Is there an effort to control workload by staggering patient arrival times?
6. Are patients received with warmth and courtesy? What provisions exist for patient and family feedback regarding treatment by staff?
7. How are patients escorted to the wards and what forms and records accompany them?

8. What care related activities come under admissions' responsibility? What routine tests are part of the admitting process, does admissions request the medical record, and is admissions responsible for notifying the attending physician of the patient's arrival?
9. Are physicians kept informed of bed occupancy levels?
10. Does admissions compile daily and weekly statistics on all activities?

Discharge Procedures

1. Who has the authority to discharge or transfer a patient and how is admissions informed?
2. What is the procedure for returning clothes and valuables?
3. Are relatives informed as early as possible and is transportation arranged for the patient? Who is responsible for being certain the patient can make the trip safely?
4. Who is responsible that the patient has received proper health care instructions and drugs if needed? What is the procedure for follow-up appointments as an outpatient?
5. What control procedures exist for the patient's medical record and other records and reports?

Admissions is a vital area for patient care and offers a substantial opportunity to provide individuals with a positive experience during their stay.

THE ROLE OF SPECIALIZED ANCILLARY SERVICES

Every patient will be subjected to numerous diagnostic tests and therapies. The hospital must provide these services on a professional basis that guarantees high quality. Good controls over quality must be present to monitor all performance with a direct feedback link to top management. A professionally performed battery of tests can do much to develop a positive emotional attitude on the part of the patient as well as provide tools for diagnosis and prescribing for the individual. All ancillary services should be audited carefully for their contribution to patient health care delivery. It is not possible to deal here with all the specialized pathology and diagnostic laboratories and therapeutic areas of hospitals. However, these internal auditing checkpoints are common to most ancillary services.

1. What procedures have been established to ensure tests, procedures, and therapies are performed by licensed and qualified staff?
2. What are the procedures for assuring that the correct service is performed

on time and properly? What procedure exists to ensure that patients do not receive a service not ordered by the physician?

3. Are the results of test procedures and therapy reported promptly and in a manner that is controlled so as to make sure the physician receives the information?

4. Are test results and films retained in an orderly fashion? Have record retention schedules been prepared and are they followed?

5. Do the various laboratories maintain logbooks that provide positive control over specimens and patients? Do the labs adequately control all processing and do the controls ensure processing on a timely basis?

6. How are drugs controlled on the wards? Do medical records reveal instances of patients' receiving drugs not ordered and of other patients' being billed for drugs never administered?

7. Is it clear to all ward and laboratory personnel and physicians how services are to be requested and reported?

8. Are personnel friendly and courteous to patients? Do patients frequently complain about the quality of care?

9. What system is used to transport patients to and from tests? Does it provide for prompt pickup and delivery?

10. Do the laboratories and therapy areas coordinate the times patients will be called for tests? Do the ancillary service areas frequently schedule their work at the same time making it difficult to get patients to all appointments?

MEDICAL RECORDS MANAGEMENT AND CONTROL

Hospitals have found the management of medical records to be a difficult task. Two types of problems have been encountered. First, systems that provide for positive control of patient medical records often prove to be restrictive and inconvenient for physicians and staff while those that provide easy access often fail to keep accurate information on where the records can be located. Second, it is extremely important that the medical record be kept accurate.

There are two reasons for this. The obvious one is for patient care. The patient's medical history must be available for review at all times and must provide an accurate and complete record of all tests and therapy results. The second reason is less important for patient care but directly affects the hospital's receiving payments from government health insurance programs. The medical record must support all charges to patients. Failure to provide this documentation can result in considerable loss of payments from the government. Internal auditors must evaluate the hospital's management and control of medical records. Below are important points to audit.

1. What procedures are there for ensuring that medical records are complete and support the patient billings? Does the system get the job done effectively and with a minimum of delays? How is this monitored?
2. What group is responsible for the management of the medical records department? Are the group members qualified to supervise the department and do they actively manage medical records systems and procedures?
3. Are medical records personnel qualified for their jobs? Are there training programs for staff?
4. Does medical records have an operating manual? Is it up to date and complete? Are the procedures adequate?
5. Are the physical facilities of the medical records department adequate? Is there sufficient equipment? Is comfortable space provided for department personnel and for physicians who come to review or complete patient records?
6. How are medical records filed? Do procedures facilitate accurate filing and quick retrieval?
7. Who is allowed access to the records and how is this enforced? Are there specific standing orders on the release of information on patients?
8. How are medical records protected from loss and destruction?
9. What reports are compiled routinely by medical records? Are there enough or too many and do the right people receive them?
10. In general, do the physicians and ward personnel believe medical records management and control procedures get the job done?

OUTPATIENT HEALTH CARE

The outpatient department (OPD) has an important role in health care delivery. Many cases do not require an inpatient visit to receive the benefits of the health care system. Again, as in the case of the inpatient, patient care must be the primary focus. All outpatient department systems and procedures must contribute directly to the patient's well-being. Internal auditors must assure themselves that outpatients receive prompt and courteous processing, starting with appointments and carrying through to payment of the bill.

Outpatient care will receive more attention in the future as efforts to contain costs lead to fewer inpatient admissions as a percentage of all patients seen. An important benefit for the hospital that provides good outpatient care will be the attraction of larger numbers of patients who will keep the inpatient beds filled in spite of lower levels of inpatient admissions. Below are checkpoints for outpatient departments.

1. Who is responsible for managing the OPD? What is the organization of the business system used by the clinics?

2. Who decides policy for the OPD and what are the policies?
3. Is there an operating manual? If so, is it up to date and complete?
4. How is the OPD staffed? How are the doctors selected? How is the supporting staff selected? Are staffing arrangements planned for flexibility to meet varying patient loads?
5. What reports does the OPD prepare and what is their distribution?
6. What is the fee schedule for the department and the doctors? How were the changes determined?
7. Are patients routinely followed up when they fail to complete prescribed treatments and make return visits? If so, with what effect?
8. How good are the physical facilities? Is there enough modern equipment in good repair? Is there enough space for patients and staff and is the area comfortable?
9. Is there good access to diagnostic labs from the OPD and are patients handled promptly and courteously by the labs? Are test results returned promptly to the OPD?
10. To what extent does the outpatient department earn its way? How are deficits (if any) made up?

Many of the audit checkpoints listed for inpatients and outpatients are interchangeable.

EMERGENCY MEDICAL CARE

There are few services as much needed or as expensive to provide as emergency medical care. The resources of the entire hospital must be available on short notice to care for the emergency needs of a community. The crisis orientation of an emergency area often fails to provide a suitable environment for even the most rudimentary of general management policies and procedures. In spite of this environment, effective but unobtrusive management systems can be designed that ensure proper patient care and attention to hospital operating policies and procedures. Internal auditors should review the emergency care area thoroughly since it may be a chronic offender against even the most thoughtfully designed management procedures.

1. How closely does the emergency room work with the OPD? Does the emergency room carry a large subacute patient care load that should be handled routinely by the OPD?
2. Are emergency room personnel assigned additional duties when the demand for emergency services is low? If so, with what result?
3. How are charges determined and accumulated? In particular, are all sup-

plies and equipment usages accounted for after emergency care has been delivered?

4. Is the emergency room properly stocked with drugs and supplies and is it well equipped?

5. Where is the emergency room located? Does it provide easy access to unloading facilities for ambulances and walk-in patients and to other areas of the hospital such as the OPD, diagnostic labs, medical records, and admissions?

6. Are emergency room personnel properly qualified and certified for such service?

7. What is the emergency room policy for extending care outside the hospital for accident victims, disasters, cardiac failure, and maternity cases? Who decides emergency room policy?

8. Does revenue generated by the emergency room support its operation?

9. What are the policies for providing information to journalists and for controlling access to patients and their records?

10. What are the procedures for protecting evidence for victims of crimes such as rape and assault? How are injured criminals handled and, in particular, gunshot wounds?

Internal auditors must assure themselves that the emergency medical care facility accomplishes the goals set for it.

PHARMACY

Hospital pharmacies contribute to the care of most patients and can provide important revenue for the institution. Physicians and patients expect prompt and accurate responses to requests for medication. Pharmacies must be equipped and prepared to formulate and deliver drugs. Pharmacy operations should have detailed written procedures that personnel must follow. Failure to provide the right drug when needed can result in immediate patient care problems and unnecessary lawsuits. Pharmacies also must be operated on a sound business basis to ensure that the hospital earns maximum revenue with minimum operating costs. Below are ten checkpoints for the pharmacy area.

1. What hospital policies and procedures provide control measures preventing members of the medical staff from abusing the privilege of writing prescriptions for narcotics and other drugs? What is the policy on prescription refills?

2. What procedures are used to control inventories of drugs and who is responsible for taking inventory? What procedures exist for disposal of ex-

pired drugs? What policies exist on approval of stocking new drugs and controlling brand proliferation?

3. What are the procedures for returning unused drugs to the pharmacy? Is unit dosage in use and is it effective? How are patient accounts credited for returned drugs? Is the process of return and crediting efficient and does it minimize the number of credits to be made?

4. What is the hospital's policy for pricing drugs? Are the pharmacy's prices in line with those of other community pharmacies? What method is used to price individual products? Are employees permitted discounts? Are late charges held to a minimum?

5. What provisions are there for emergency drugs for the wards and emergency room? How are they controlled?

6. Is the pharmacy conveniently located for outpatients? Is there a convenient waiting area?

7. What drugs and solutions are manufactured by the pharmacy? How is the production process controlled? Is up to date equipment used and are all processes efficient? Are solutions spot checked for contamination?

8. What are the procedures for cleaning the pharmacy? Who performs the routine janitorial work? Is the work performed in a manner that avoids contaminating drug inventories? How are drugs safeguarded from all maintenance and housekeeping personnel who may have routine access to the pharmacy?

9. What agreements, if any, exist with other pharmacies in the community for emergency prescription service?

10. What are the procedures for handling cash receipts? What types of reports on activities are prepared? How many, how often, and who receives them? Do the reports fairly represent the pharmacies' performance?

A properly operating pharmacy is crucial for hospitals. Internal auditors should make thorough operations reviews of all phases of pharmacy operation to assure the administration that patient care and hospital interests are being met properly.

OPERATIONS AUDITING IN OTHER PATIENT-RELATED AREAS

Operations auditing may be applied to virtually any patient care area of the hospital. Internal auditors eventually must evaluate the entire hospital to be certain all departments and operating areas are contributing to the institution's goals. Additional areas related to patient care are: central supply services, dietetics, nutrition and food service, housekeeping, social services, volunteers, chaplain service, and engineering and maintenance. Two extremely important areas not covered here but that should be reviewed in detail are nursing service and ward management. It is obvious that hospitals are indeed complex organizations with many varying types of departments and activities, all of which must contribute to patient care.

CONCLUSION

Internal auditors have an important responsibility for verifying that the hospital provides the means for satisfactory patient care. While auditors cannot evaluate the quality of care patients receive from physicians, nurses, and paraprofessionals, they can verify that the hospital has provided basic policies and procedures for delivering good service. Internal auditors must assure administrators and governing boards that the hospital is providing an outstanding operating environment for physicians, patients, and support staff.

Chapter 12

Operations Auditing of Hospital Support Areas

There are many nonpatient care activities in hospitals that have important secondary effects on patient care. Chapter 11 outlined avenues for applying operations auditing to hospital functions directly responsible for patient care. All of these areas are dependent to some extent on other hospital supporting activities for personnel, safety, purchasing, and information. Hospitals cannot provide good health care without adequate assistance from these support functions. Internal auditors must evaluate all areas of the institution that may have an indirect impact on patient care. Depending on size and location, hospitals will have a wide range of departments and functions. Six departments found in most hospitals are safety and security, personnel, public relations, purchasing, data processing, and laundry. These departments and functions demonstrate the diverse hospital activities that can be subjected to operations audits. Below, ten audit checkpoints are provided for each of the six departments. Those listed for one department often can be applied to many others.

SAFETY AND SECURITY

Safety has become a national issue and employee, patient, and visitor safety has become increasingly more important to the Joint Commission on Hospital Accreditation. Hospitals must be aware of needs for safety because of their unique role in society. Security is a second major concern. The importance of good security often is not appreciated until a crime against the hospital or one of its employees, patients, or visitors occurs. The extent of security measures depends on location and past experience. Hospitals in relatively crime-free areas, however, cannot overlook minimum security needs.

1. What written procedures exist for safety and security? Are they complete and do they comply with existing laws and regulations?

2. Who is responsible for safety and security? Does the existing organization aid in achieving safety and security goals?
3. What are the hospital's plans for evacuation in the event of fire or other disaster? What procedures exist for keeping track of patients as they are moved about within the hospital?
4. Does the hospital have a policy of requiring patients, visitors, and employees to complete accident reports?
5. Are there safety training programs, including fire fighting training? Is there a program of regular inspection for safety hazards?
6. How does the hospital control access to all buildings and all rooms? Does the plan, in fact, control access and is it followed?
7. What are the procedures for reporting loss, damage to, or theft of property of the hospital, patients, visitors, and employees? Do they appear effective?
8. How safe are the hospital's grounds and parking lots? Are they properly lighted and patrolled? Is there an escort service for female employees, visitors, and patients if requested?
9. Does the hospital have an active program of crime prevention? Are keys to rooms carefully controlled? Are pieces of equipment engraved with control numbers? Are supplies carefully monitored with attention directed to drugs, syringes, and other items of value to drug addicts?
10. Are hospital security personnel properly trained, equipped, and supervised? Are there enough personnel?

Safety and security issues pertain to all areas of the hospital, all functions, all patients, and all employees. Internal auditors must be alert for such problems in audit projects.[1]

PERSONNEL ADMINISTRATION

There may be no other single function in hospitals that can have as great of an impact on employee morale and performance as a poor program of personnel administration.[2] Hospital personnel departments should perform the following functions: recruiting, employee orientation, labor relations, terminations and grievances, administration of wages and salaries, maintenance of employee records, training programs, and employee evaluations. Much literature on hospital personnel administration exists. Internal auditors of large hospitals with relatively large personnel departments should audit each of the above functions and any others separately. Auditors in hospitals with small personnel departments probably can review the entire department at one time. Regardless of the exact methodology, internal auditors should be able to design comprehensive audit programs for the personnel administration department that will yield important findings for the hospital's management. Ten sets of the more important checkpoints are provided below.[3,4,5]

1. Have the organization, authority, and responsibilities of the personnel department been defined? Have policies been written and are they complete and up to date?[6]
2. Are all members of the personnel department's staff qualified for their jobs? Is there enough staff, space, and equipment?
3. What is the attitude of the hospital's administration toward personnel management, organized labor, wage and salary administration, training programs, and all other phases of personnel administration? Is the administration supportive and generally prepared to provide the resources required by personnel management programs?
4. What reports does personnel generate routinely? For example, what is the hospital's turnover rate? Is the rate broken down by job title? What is the average time required for recruiting for various job titles? How much training is needed?
5. Are all jobs properly described? Are wages and salaries set with skill levels in mind? Do employees believe the hospital's wages, salaries, and fringe benefits are acceptable? How do they compare with other nearby hospitals and industries? How are staffing levels determined and by whom?
6. How actively does the personnel department recruit nurses, technicians, secretaries, and clerks? How are applicants interviewed and screened? Who is responsible for making the employment decision?[7]
7. How active a role does the personnel department have in maintaining and improving employee morale? Are employees allowed to feed back complaints and suggestions? How does the administration respond to this feedback? Does the hospital have a news publication that is distributed to all employees?
8. How adequate are training, orientation, employee evaluation, and personnel record management programs? Are there adequate procedures and are they followed?[8]
9. Are employee attitudes surveyed and, if so, with what result? Has top management been responsive to real or perceived employee needs and wants?
10. What role does the personnel department play in forecasting needs and in preparing plans to meet them?

From this list, the breadth of the functions of a personnel department, its impact on the hospital's ability to meet its goals, and the degree of difficulty internal auditors will have in performing productive operations audits can be visualized. To add to the challenge is the newness of the concept of auditing personnel management. The administration of the department will be sensitive to such a review and all audit personnel should be cautioned not to provoke unnecessary alarm or skepticism during the project. Furthermore, because of the confidential nature of many of the records, auditors must take every precaution not to compromise their confidentiality.

PUBLIC RELATIONS

Public relations and communications for hospitals have grown in importance as society increasingly has questioned the health care industry. Hospital administrators must develop good public relations and communication programs.[9] The responsibility for public relations begins with hospital directors. They will find their attitudes reflected throughout the hospital: whatever their position, it is likely to become the general attitude for the entire institution.[10] Directors therefore must have positive attitudes and by example set the general attitude for the whole hospital. An institution with an overall good administrative attitude should have a good image to portray to the public, and it also will develop in its employees a positive attitude toward patients and health care that will compliment management's efforts.

Internal auditors may find auditing a function such as public relations strange, and admittedly it is; however, operations auditing can be applied to all functions to some extent and to the degree that this can be done, the unit can benefit. As usual, internal auditors planning to evaluate public relations and communications must prepare by reviewing available literature. They will have to be resourceful when designing audit programs for public relations because the final product is difficult to measure. Below are ten checkpoints for a public relations and communications audit program.

1. How is the function organized and staffed? What policies and procedures have been established, by whom, and are they in writing?
2. Have goals been established and standards set to measure performance where possible? Are the standards in fact measurable?[11]
3. Are the goals of the program compatible with those of the hospital? What provisions are there for reviewing public relations goals and hospital goals to ensure they will continue to complement each other?
4. What patterns of communication have been established between top management and public relations personnel? Are the patterns adequate? Do they provide for accurate and timely information?
5. Is there overall planning for the public relations program?

6. Have contingency plans been prepared and agreed upon for handling unusual events such as attacks by the media or special interests?
7. What provision has been made for feedback from the public and employees? Is the information acted on?
8. Are files maintained of clippings from newspapers and journals? Are they used to key new ideas on presenting the hospital's health care story?
9. What efforts are made to improve employee attitudes toward patient care and the hospital? How effective are the existing methods of communicating with employees?[12]
10. Does the general atmosphere of the hospital bespeak an effective public relations attitude on the part of the administration?

Internal auditors in hospitals with especially poor track records for public relations and communications may find some assistance by sampling public and employee opinions. If the problem appears serious enough, the internal auditor may want to recommend that consultants analyze the situation. Hospitals no longer can ignore the need for good public relations. A large part of the current travail in which hospitals find themselves is the direct result of neglecting to sell the merits of the health care industry.

PURCHASING

After auditing public relations, the internal auditor will be pleased to return to more familiar ground. The purchasing function often is subjected to financial and compliance type auditing as well as operations audits. Operations auditing is stressed because it offers the hospital maximum opportunity for improvement. The purchasing function is second only to a hospital's salary and wages in fiscal importance. Hospitals can lose large sums from a poorly performing purchasing system. A vast array of literature on purchasing exists. Below are ten sets of checkpoints.

1. What is purchasing's organization? Is it staffed adequately with qualified employees? Are its systems and procedures documented? Are they adequate? Is purchasing independent of receiving and accounts payable?[13,14]
2. Is the purchasing department and its operations organized to promote efficient and effective processing of orders? How does the volume of orders and their dollar value correspond with staffing and paper processing costs?[15]
3. What procedures exist for authorizing purchases? Are they adequate and are they followed? Has the administration defined the purchasing department's powers and responsibilities and does it have effective means for controlling the department?

4. Are purchasing's facilities adequate? Is there adequate space for receiving and interviewing vendors? Are there adequate records and forms? How are they safeguarded from loss?[16]

5. Does the purchasing department exhibit leadership in keeping the hospital stocked at reasonable levels at minimum costs and with few supply outages? Does the hospital participate in group purchasing? Are competitive bids used? Are new vendors sought out? Are orders submitted so as to take advantage of quantity discounts? What controls exist over product proliferation?[17]

6. Does the purchasing department exhibit a service orientation to other hospital departments? If purchasing is completely centralized, how do units such as pathology, pharmacy, and central supply view the purchasing department's functioning? Are communications with purchasing good?

7. What reports does purchasing routinely prepare and what are their distribution? Are the reports timely and accurate and do they provide meaningful management information? Do the reports reveal the cost effectiveness of the purchasing department?

8. What procedures exist for emergency ordering? Is the privilege used frequently and, if so, why?

9. Do written purchasing policies exist and have they been communicated to all hospital personnel directly and indirectly related to the function? Are there policies for vendors and have they been communicated? Do the policies cover points such as purchases for employees, gifts from vendors, relationships with departments, receiving, and accounts payable? Do the policies help ensure a high level of integrity by all concerned?

10. Do the internal checks on the purchasing department provide good control of paperwork, orders, bids, discounts, vendors, and reorder points? Do the controls operate efficiently? What actions are taken to resolve problems such as duplicate orders or shipments, credits, purchase orders unmatched with receiving reports, and damaged or otherwise unacceptable goods? Does purchasing learn from its problems with vendors and other departments? From its own problems?

The role of purchasing in hospitals is important and can help greatly in holding down the rising costs of medical care.

ELECTRONIC DATA PROCESSING

There is perhaps no other recent innovation that has greater promise nor promises greater confusion that the application of computers to the health care industry. The range of application has few limits in either health care delivery or administration. Increased operating complexity often results when hospitals acquire electronic data processing. This requires sound management of the systems in order to gain the benefits they offer, including lower costs. Lack of attention to managing data processing systems can result in increased costs and eventually inferior results in all hospital areas.

The field of internal auditing has been challenged to provide good operations audit coverage and literature on the subject now exists. Hospital internal auditors will find operational reviews of computerized systems a challenge that can be met only by careful preparation. Below are ten general checkpoints that must be included in any audit of a data processing system.

1. How is the data processing area staffed? Are the director and staff properly qualified? Are training programs adequate? Has internal auditing planned for effective uses of commercially available computer auditing software packages?[18]

2. Does the data processing function provide the hospital's administration with timely, accurate, and useful information that effectively and efficiently supports the decision-making process—a key performance measure?[19]

3. Do systems that have been implemented actually perform in the manner planned? How do the costs and actual benefits compare with plan? Are differences carefully isolated and evaluated? Are the differences the result of poor planning, poor performance, or both?

4. What is the relationship of the data processing department to the rest of the hospital? Is it independent or does it report to a department such as finance? It is recommended the data processing function report directly to the hospital director.

5. Electronic data processing requires the design of very complicated systems and procedures. Is there adequate documentation that is accurate and up to date?[20] This is a frequent problem area that cannot be neglected without negative consequences.

6. Have clear goals and objectives been established for data processing? Have standards of performance been set and communicated? Are the standards measurable? A function that is this complicated and expensive and has such a broad impact requires a thorough continuing management oversight process.

7. Is there sufficient short-term, intermediate, and long-range planning? Planning covers the entire range of operations from improving schedules and utilization, to preparing for major changes in hospital operations, to implementing new programs, to complete replacement of existing hardware and software as new technology in health care and computers emerges.[21]

8. What reports are prepared routinely for top management on data processing operations? Are they accurate and of use? Do they enable management to evaluate and control the function?

9. Is top management able to communicate effectively with EDP personnel, do the executives understand EDP, and do they contribute actively to planning, design, and evaluation of data processing systems? Does top management appear to be uninformed about computers and their operation and generally avoid dealing with EDP personnel?

10. Has adequate attention been given to the dehumanizing effects of computerization on patients and employees?

Hospitals using computers in any manner regardless whether they are related to patient care, administration, or both must review all EDP applications carefully and completely. Internal auditors are suited ideally to make these reviews as few hospital staff members will have a broader conception of the total institution and the effects of computerization. Hospital administrators must be certain internal auditing is prepared to perform operations evaluations of all data processing. Significant savings are provided by improving existing systems and by avoiding the use of expensive consultants who frequently are brought in to solve problems.

LAUNDRY

Hospitals must handle the cleaning of large volumes of soiled and contaminated bed linen, robes, gowns, towels, blankets, and other reusable cloth items. For large hospitals, the volume may reach many thousands of pounds a month. Efficient and economical laundry handling is essential to keeping adequate supplies of clean items on hand at all times at a reasonable cost. Internal auditors must evaluate hospital procedures for handling laundry by using operations auditing methods. Auditors must be alert for procedures or problems that add unnecessary costs or produce unsanitary processing and missed opportunities for improvement. In hospitals that contract for laundry services, auditors must evaluate the terms of the contract and the quality of the service to ensure that the institution is receiving good results at a reasonable cost. Below are ten sets of audit checkpoints on laundry handling.

1. Is the laundry adequately staffed? Does labor turnover appear to disrupt operations?

2. What has been the laundry's safety record? How many injuries have been reported? Are there any obvious safety hazards? Is the laundry clean and adequately lighted and ventilated?

3. Are the employees supervised properly? Does the laundry manager report to management on operations? Does the manager communicate freely with all hospital areas that generate laundry as to needs and problems?

4. How well is the laundry equipped? Is the equipment in good operating condition? Who is responsible for maintaining it?

5. How are inventory records of linen in storerooms and in circulation maintained? How often is it inventoried physically? What is the expected life of linen in service? What costs are associated with repair and replacement? Is there an adequate amount of inventory, too little, too much?

6. How is laundry processed? How is contaminated, stained, and infected linen washed? Are detergents suited to water hardness and do they contribute to pollution? What is the usual processing time required to have linen back in service?

7. How do operating costs compare with commercial laundry services? Is accurate cost information available for comparison? Are utilities used by the laundry metered separately?

8. How is laundry transported? How are soiled items delivered to the laundry? How is contaminated laundry marked and separated from regular laundry? What records are kept of laundry received and delivered?

9. How is damaged linen detected and repaired? Is there a sewing room for repairs? What other services are offered by the sewing room? Is the sewing room equipped properly?

10. What is the overall quality of the laundry's service? Do nursing personnel believe the laundry service is good?

A good operations audit will be most beneficial to the laundry. Patient care can be affected directly by poor laundry processing and hospital costs increased by uneconomical laundry operations.

CONCLUSION

Internal auditing has a responsibility for operations reviews of all hospital activities that support patient care goals. The internal auditing approach provides in-depth operations reviews of the hospital's many diverse departments. Poorly run support departments can produce short- and long-run problems if top management is not kept informed systematically of actual operations. Independent operations reviews have the benefit of spotting wastes and inefficiencies that have been accepted or have gone unrecognized by department managers. Hospital directors must be certain internal auditors conduct thorough operations audits of all patient care support departments.

NOTES

1. D. A. Tovell, "Successful Safety Evaluation," *Internal Auditor*, December 1974, pp. 36–44.

2. N. Morris, "Auditing the Personnel Function," *Internal Auditor*, April 1975, p. 26.

3. Victor Z. Brink, James A. Cashin, and Herbert Witt, *Modern Internal Auditing: An Operational Approach* (New York: The Ronald Press Company, 1973), pp. 320–324.

4. Dale L. Flesher, *Operations Auditing in Hospitals* (Lexington, Mass.: Lexington Books, 1976), pp. 79–84.

5. Roy A. Lindberg and Theodore Cohn, *Operations Auditing* (New York: American Management Association, 1972), pp. 230–236.

6. B. J. Hall, *Auditing the Modern Hospital* (Englewood Cliffs, N.J.: Prentice-Hall, Inc., 1977), p. 200.

7. Ibid., pp. 202–203.

8. American Hospital Association, *Internal Control and Internal Auditing in Hospitals* (Chicago: American Hospital Association, 1969), p. 9.

9. C. A. Oliphant, *Public Relations for Health Care Management* (Cleveland, Tenn.: Hospital Publications, Inc., 1975), p. v.

10. Ibid., p. 18.

11. Ibid., p. 54.

12. J. F. Milne and N. W. Chaplin, ed., *Modern Hospital Management* (London: The Institute of Hospital Administration, Ltd., 1969), p. 495.

13. R. N. Gilbert, "Operational Auditing," *Hospital Financial Management*, August 1977, p. 31.

14. Ray E. Brown and Richard L. Johnson, *Hospitals Visualized* (Chicago: American College of Hospital Administrators, 1957), p. 119.

15. Lindberg, op. cit., p. 194.

16. Brink, op. cit., pp. 140–141.

17. Flesher, op. cit., p. 99.

18. M. R. Moore, "Computer Auditing in the 1970's," *Internal Auditor*, June 1974, p. 40.

19. H. M. Sollenberger and A. A. Arens, "Systems Control and the Post-Completion Systems Audit," *Internal Auditor*, April 1973, p. 24.

20. J. J. Cortey-Merrifield, "The Implications of EDP Documentation for the Internal Auditor," *Internal Auditor*, February 1977, pp. 38–42.

21. Lindberg, op. cit., p. 164.

Chapter 13

Financial and Compliance Auditing in Hospitals

Financial and compliance auditing always have been important parts of the internal auditing function. Until the 1940s, for the most part they were the only activities internal auditors performed. The benefits that can be derived from these types of audits are fewer than those of operations audits, primarily because the auditor does not evaluate the operations of a department as a process within a larger system or top management's role in overseeing the department. Financial auditing is concerned with the adequacy of the internal control of cash, accounting, assets, receipts, disbursements, payroll, billing, and any other elements that impact on hospital finances. Compliance auditing involves all activities that have written procedures.[1] Internal auditors review the adequacy of the written procedures in terms of internal control and then assess the extent to which employees comply with them.

Closely related to financial and compliance auditing, and of concern to all hospitals, is fraud. Most administrators associate auditors with the detection of fraud; unfortunately, this is not correct. Internal auditors are responsible for exercising due professional care in performing their function. Due care implies internal auditors must be alert for possible wrongdoings by anyone from top management on down.[2] This basically means internal auditors must track down every questionable finding and ultimately determine its cause.[3] This will include both findings auditors uncover and those brought to their attention.

The *Standards for the Professional Practice of Internal Auditing* state that internal auditors cannot give assurance that noncompliance or irregularities do not exist. The department's management must assume full responsibility for fraud that occurs on transactions not included in the audit sample. It must be added that fraud is difficult to uncover and to guard against.[4,5] There are no economical systems that stop all fraud. One of the best methods of prevention is a continuing process of employee education that makes all personnel security conscious.[6] Fraud awareness programs in hospitals can make a definite contribution to controlling the risks of embezzlement and theft of the institution's assets.

This chapter covers many of the more important hospital areas where effective internal and financial controls are required as safeguards against needless losses.[7] The emphasis is on financial and compliance auditing, but the good internal auditor always will be alert to the need for future operations audits. Only the operations audit will evaluate the department's contribution to the hospital's overall goals. Any financial area can accomplish its work effectively with an abundance of good internal controls, but the cost may be much higher than is acceptable.

ACCOUNTS PAYABLE

All hospitals must expend funds for supplies, equipment, and salaries. Payroll control will be discussed later. The purchase of supplies and equipment requires a process of financial control to assure prompt, authorized, and accurate payments are made to vendors and that the materials paid for have been received in good order. Hospitals can lose funds to embezzlers unnecessarily by paying for materials not received. Hospitals also may expend funds unnecessarily when they do not take advantage of discounts for prompt payment. As can be seen from the ten sets of audit checkpoints below, a good accounts payable system needs many internal controls.

1. What procedures are used to control accounts payable? Are requests for purchases entered into the purchasing system at the earliest possible time? Is there a controlling ledger? Are only purchase transactions recorded? How does the system control against double payments?
2. What is the frequency with which payments are made to vendors? Is there a period of accumulation before preparing a check to pay multiple invoices or are many small checks issued at additional cost?
3. When the person authorized to approve disbursements signs the checks or vouchers, is supporting documentation available for review? Are receiving notices provided? Have all invoice prices, extensions, and footings been checked for accuracy? Are checks ever made out to employees or cash? Who mails the checks after they are signed?
4. Are vendor discounts taken advantage of? Are they paid near the last day of the discount's availability so as to permit the hospital use of the funds a few additional days?
5. How are credit memos handled? Do they become the responsibility of the accounting department? How are orders and payments controlled on blanket authorizations? How are advance payments controlled?
6. Are all accounts paid within vendor time limits? This will require preparing a schedule that ages accounts payable. Are delinquent accounts reviewed and resolved?

7. Is there a significant number of deficiencies in accounts payable? If so, the auditor should consider confirming a sample of all vendors, regardless of whether or not hospital records indicate an active accounts payable balance.
8. How are records of requisitions, orders, vouchers, and disbursements maintained? What is their retention period? Are they cross-referenced so as to permit inquiries by vendor, purchase order, or disbursement?
9. What organizational relationships exist among purchasing, receiving, accounting, and check signing? Are they independent of each other? What are the paper flows to and from each area and what are their responsibilities? For example, which area receives invoices—purchasing or accounting? Are procedures used in conformance with the governing board's guidelines?
10. Are good internal controls evident in each department or are many functions performed by a few persons in some departments?

Many of these audit checkpoints can be applied to other types of payables such as travel expenses, financing through loans and notes, and insurance payments.

ACCOUNTS RECEIVABLE

Large hospitals will have many millions of dollars involved in pending payments from patients and third-party payors. Good internal control is a key element in managing accounts receivable. Internal control prevents fraud and guards against errors. Accounts receivable are subject to several types of manipulation that can produce illegal benefits for employees and their friends. Balances can be reduced or unapplied payments posted to accounts either to pay off a bill or even as a refund. While fraud is a valid concern, the effective management of hospital accounts receivable often can be difficult. A lack of good internal control can make the task virtually impossible without an overwhelming number of daily operating problems. Ten sets of audit points are listed below.

1. What policies have been developed to deal with decisions on credit, referrals of patient accounts to collection agencies, and bad debts? Are they reasonable and are they followed? Who is authorized to approve these types of decisions? Are personnel responsible for approving credit denied access to cash? What policies and procedures exist for unapplied payments?

2. Does the organization of the accounts receivable section, credit department, cashier, and collection department promote good internal control? Are employees of these sections restricted from working in the other areas even during lunch breaks and absences? How are records safeguarded from unauthorized access? What provisions are there for sharing or lending records?

3. What type of controlling account or ledger is used for accounts receivable? Are the accounts receivable reconciled on a regular basis?

4. Do the types, size, and aging of accounts receivable and bad debt write-offs resemble national averages?

5. How are cash receipts posted to individual accounts and are they reconciled to total receipts?

6. In what form are patient accounts maintained? What detail is available on charges and payments?

7. How often and in what manner are charges posted? What internal controls exist that ensure all charges are posted and correctly? Are there many late charges? Is a total bill available to the patient at departure?

8. How are credit balances controlled? What are the policies and procedures for refunding credit balances to the patient? Who authorizes the refunds? Are there enough credit balances to affect reporting of accounts receivable materially? If so, credit balances should be placed in a separate account.

9. What reports are prepared routinely and what is their distribution? Are all exceptions reported? Are accounts receivable aging schedules prepared that cover aging by date of discharge, by date of last payment, and by area of payment responsibility starting with the discharge date? What reports are prepared on unapplied payments?

10. Is confirmation of accounts receivable performed? This may be a standard step of the certified public accounting firm's annual audit. This process will help determine whether patients' payments have been applied properly to their accounts.

Internal auditors should conduct a thorough review of the systems and procedures that make up the internal controls for the accounts receivable function. Many risks and inefficiencies can be uncovered and opportunities often exist for redesigning portions of the systems and procedures to improve performance and reduce costs. Of great importance in all financial auditing is the degree of employee compliance. This becomes increasingly important with expansions in the size of the systems and number of employees. All instances of noncompliance must be documented carefully. While noncompliance findings can result in disciplinary measures, they also can be used to analyze the reasons why the noncompliance was not uncovered by the daily operating procedures. Auditors should not overlook the possibility that the written procedures have not dealt successfully with the problem discovered and that the employee was left with no alternative other than to develop a procedure that worked.

PAYROLL

A hospital's payroll is its largest single operating expense. Many millions of dollars in salaries are required even for modest-sized hospitals. A good payroll system can operate effectively and often go unnoticed by employees or can be a frequent source of conflict when personnel are paid improperly or not at all. Hospital salaries and wages must conform to the Fair Labor Standards Act, as must parts of the payroll system. Payrolls must be documented adequately, with records retained for specified periods. Fraud again is a concern, with possible additional payments made to some employees or checks made out to ones who do not exist, with the check picked up and cashed by a member of the payroll staff or of another department.

The proper functioning of the payroll department is crucial in terms of getting out an accurate payroll on time. This requires a carefully designed and closely supervised system with tight internal controls. Below are ten sets of audit checkpoints for an effective payroll audit program.

1. What records are used to control payroll? How are pay scales checked for accuracy? How are payroll calculations checked, including computations of overtime, holiday pay, and call time? How and for how long are records retained? How are payroll deductions authorized and reported to employees? What records are used to document employees' receipt of pay?
2. How are payroll checking accounts controlled? Are they regularly reconciled by employees other than payroll's? Are payroll employees properly bonded? Does the hospital use multiple payroll checking accounts to save time on reconciliations? Multiple accounts will allow reconciliations of individual payroll periods. Reconciliations can be timed to permit most, if not all, checks to be accounted for.
3. What internal controls are in evidence? Are the various payroll steps distributed among employees? Are employees rotated on jobs on a regular basis? What provisions are there to avoid using employees of one department to fill in for absences or lunch hours in other departments and thus permit possible tampering with records? Are blank payroll checks safeguarded properly? Are checks prenumbered? Who is responsible for approving or signing the payroll and the checks? Do the steps taken by the person in charge guard effectively against error and fraud?

4. What is the procedure for distributing payroll checks and cash? How are employees identified? How are unclaimed payroll checks and payments handled? Does a department other than payroll resolve the exceptions? What procedure is there for mailing out income tax statements? Does the procedure secure the statements from tampering? Who is responsible for mailing checks and statements? How are returned checks and statements handled?

5. Who is responsible for authorizing hiring, pay scales, and overtime? Are there sufficient records by employee to document hiring levels and raises? What forms must new hires complete? Are W-4 forms completed regularly?

6. What types of time records are kept? Are they accurate? Do supervisors monitor employees closely to make sure times reported are correct? What records are maintained for vacations and sick leave?

7. Do the payroll systems and procedures appear to be efficient and accomplish the function at a minimum of cost? Do they promote accuracy? Does the system handle emergency payroll situations effectively?

8. Are payroll disbursements made on time? Are all time records and other documents received on schedule from all departments? What electronic data processing applications exist?

9. How is the confidentiality of the payroll records safeguarded? Do payroll employees avoid discussing records with others? Are records disposed of in a manner that safeguards confidentiality?

10. What reports and analyses are prepared routinely of payroll matters and what is their distribution? Are quarterly tax reports prepared on time and deposits made?

From audit to audit, the program should be reexamined with an eye for finding approaches that may uncover new problems and deficiencies and for exploring all changes in procedure that have occurred since the last audit.

CASH RECEIPTS

Hospitals often handle large sums of cash payments by patients. The management of cash receipts requires sound internal control and supervision to guard against errors and fraud. Cash represents a high risk because it is vulnerable to theft. Employees taking cash need worry only about covering up its disappearance, unlike fraud in purchasing or accounts receivable in which the employee must convert transactions into cash or something of value. Accounting for cash also can be difficult unless effective operating procedures are used. Errors represent real and immediate dollar losses and problems that require resolution.

Internal auditors must be thorough in their reviews of cash receipts and insist on suitable internal controls and procedures.[8] The ten sets of audit checkpoints below cover important aspects of reviewing cash receipts.

1. Is the custody of cash separated from those responsible for cash receipt records and reporting? Cashiers must be responsible only for receiving cash, not accounting for it. Are all employees properly bonded? How are new employees screened to avoid hiring persons with obvious problems in their work history?
2. Is a minimum number of employees involved with handling cash? How are absences and lunch hours covered?
3. Is cash received centrally? If not, are remote locations properly staffed, equipped, and controlled? Is cash adequately protected physically? Are daily deposits made intact?
4. Are employees required to rotate jobs and to take vacations?
5. If the hospital routinely cashes checks, is an imprest fund used? Are the procedures associated with the fund followed closely?
6. Are mail payments opened and listed by personnel other than the cashier's office or accounting? Are reports of the mail receipts provided to persons who ultimately can check the amounts deposited? Are checks restrictively endorsed at once?
7. Are cash registers used for over-the-counter payments? Is the cash drawer balanced against the internal tape? Are prenumbered receipts used? What provision is there for multiple cashiers?
8. Is the bank deposit slip returned to someone other than the cashier's office or accounting? Is an armored car service used to transfer cash?
9. How are cash receipts for interest, dividends, sale of scrap, rents, and all other nonpatient care revenues handled? Are they reported separately from patient fee revenue?
10. Does the institution receive payments for physicians and other health care professionals not paid by the hospital?

Internal auditors should examine top management's handling and control of cash to verify that cash balances are put to good use. Auditors also may reduce the time public accountants devote to auditing cash receipts in favor of using the time elsewhere more productively.

UNCOLLECTABLE PATIENT ACCOUNTS

An audit of uncollected patient accounts and related systems and procedures may seem at first to be an unnecessary review. After all, why invest time in a review of records known not to be expected to generate any funds for the hospital? However, there is much that needs to be audited to ensure patient accounts written off as bad debts in fact are uncollectable. A secondary aspect is to analyze why the bad debts are incurred. The analysis may lead to changes in screening and admitting procedures.

1. Are accounts that are written off as bad debts adequately documented as to all efforts at collection? Are all policies and procedures followed? How rigorous are they? Do they permit an unnecessarily high level of uncollected accounts to be written off? Were the policies approved by the governing board?

2. Are bad debt write-offs authorized by a position that exercises control over the process?

3. How are bad debts reported and accounted for? How are the records maintained and for how long?

4. Is a sample of bad debts confirmed to assure that collection efforts are rigorous enough and that the debts are not abused?

5. Are uncollected accounts referred to a collection agency? Are these referrals controlled by a separate account?

6. Is the collection agency making a reasonable effort on all accounts or does it concentrate on the easier ones? What impact does the collection agency's efforts have on community relations?

7. What has been learned from the hospital's uncollectable accounts experience? Is there an indication policies and procedures need to be changed?

8. What impact does the hospital's screening procedure have on uncollectable accounts? Does the screening include verification of insurance coverage and credit? Does the hospital have adequate financial counseling for patients?

9. Are the credit, collections, and counseling areas adequately staffed by qualified personnel?

10. What is the hospital's policy on patients who return for care with account balances owed from prior visits?

A thorough audit of bad debts may yield many insights into preventing unnecessary losses and provide information on which to base recommendations for changes in policies and procedures elsewhere in the hospital.

INVENTORIES OF SUPPLIES AND EQUIPMENT

Hospitals have sizable investments in supply inventories and equipment. To be certain they invest no more resources than necessary and yet avoid operating problems requires records that are accurate and planned carefully. The systems and procedures used must be reviewed to ensure maximum control at minimum expense. Thorough internal audits of hospital inventories and inventory procedures can yield substantial savings and reduced risks. Inventory procedures and internal audit checkpoints are available from many sources, and several should be consulted before completing an audit program.

1. Does the hospital have a central receiving area that checks in all supplies and equipment? Is central receiving independent of purchasing, accounting, and ordering departments? Are copies of receiving slips placed in the hands of the person approving disbursements? What control exists over free samples of drugs and supplies? How are narcotics controlled and does the control meet federal standards?

2. Are perpetual inventory records maintained on all major classes of supplies by personnel other than the storeroom's? Are electronic data processing applications appropriate?

3. Have inventory reorder points been established for all supplies? Are the reorder amounts reasonable? Do they take advantage of quantity discounts? How often do stock outages occur?

4. What controls exist over the total number and types of supplies stocked? Is there an unwarranted proliferation of items? Is there stock on hand that no longer is used?

5. What are the procedures for distributing supplies? What documents are used? Do the procedures require proper authorizations? Is adequate information provided to permit the storeroom to bill the right patient or department? What is the procedure for pricing?

6. With what frequency are physical inventories taken? What are the procedures for taking the inventory? Who supervises the inventory counting process? Are spot checks made of the accuracy of counts by disinterested employees or internal auditors? Who may authorize a change in perpetual inventory records? How are shortages and overages reported and to whom?

7. How are supplies stored? Is there enough space that is properly climate controlled and free from spoilage by water or pests? Is the area clean? Are supplies stored in an orderly manner? What condition are the supplies in? Are supplies with limited shelf lives rotated carefully to ensure that none expire before use? How are supplies secured from theft and fire?

8. Is there adequate documentation on purchases of equipment? Are warranties, maintenance agreements, and leases controlled adequately?

9. How is the equipment controlled? Are inventory numbers assigned individual pieces of equipment and affixed securely? How often is equipment

inventoried? What procedures are followed and who supervises the process?

10. What are the hospital's policies on equipment depreciation? Is depreciation properly claimed on equipment?

Effective internal control of supply and equipment inventories can yield many benefits for hospitals. Internal auditors must be certain the institutions control and manage their inventories properly.

PATIENT BILLING

Patient billing systems are as numerous as hospitals. Large hospitals generally have come to rely on fully computerized or at least computer-assisted systems while smaller hospitals must rely on manual methods with varying levels of sophistication. All billing systems have in common the compiling of an accurate and timely record of all charges for all patients. To the extent the systems fail in this or succeed at excessive cost, hospitals lose resources. Internal auditors, when designing audit programs for hospital billing systems, must be resourceful to do a thorough job without requiring an excessive amount of time. Below are ten sets of audit checkpoints that demonstrate how financial and compliance auditing may be blended with operations auditing.

1. Do the medical records support the charges to patients? Are there records or reports for all laboratory tests and are there physician and technician notes for all professional services rendered and billed?

2. How are business records maintained? Is the system economical and does it promote accuracy and efficiency? What use is made of microfilm? What records retention schedules have been prepared and are they reasonable? Are records retrieved quickly when requested? How secure are the records from damage, loss, and search by unauthorized personnel?

3. Are patient billings reviewed routinely for obvious problems and errors? The process used should be expected to spot obvious billing errors that appear out of the ordinary. Are there numerous late charges?

4. What procedure is used to determine hospital charges and how often are existing charges adjusted and new ones added? Are there adequate cost finding studies? Do charges comply with cost containment guidelines?

5. Are charges compiled by revenue centers so as to permit comparisons with operating costs?

6. What controls are used to assure that all chargeable supplies and services are billed to the patient? Are inventories of supplies controlled to permit accounting for sales and unexplained shrinkages? Are billing system

forms designed thoughtfully and, when appropriate, controlled by pre-numbering? What methods are used in batching and batch control?

7. What are the procedures for computing, checking, and entering contractual adjustments on patient accounts?

8. What is the procedure for billing the hospital room rate to the patient? Is the record used to prepare the billing reliable? Does the procedure allow for instances such as a patient transfer to an intensive care unit and return to the ward on the same day?

9. Does the billing system provide for adequate detailed and summary reporting? Are detailed reports of all charges sorted in a manner to permit inquiry? Do summary reports provide management useful information? What use is made of them?

10. Is there a continuing system for auditing at least a sample of medical records for supporting documentation for charges? This is an especially important process for hospitals that have large patient populations with Medicare and Medicaid coverage.

These checkpoints will require the internal auditor to become completely familiar with the central billing system and all hospital areas generating charges. There is little doubt a thorough audit of the billing system will require careful planning to avoid spending excessive time. All of the system must be explored eventually for correct operation. Time availability may require a major audit of the central system combined with appraisals of several areas that generate a large volume of charges. During the year, spot audits can be made of the central system and other areas that produce charges. A continuous audit program such as this has the added benefit of keeping more personnel and areas alert to the needs of the billing system.

CONCLUSION

Hospital fiscal systems must be designed to provide maximum internal control and compliance at a minimum of expense. This is a challenging requirement that internal auditors are prepared to help fulfill. Financial and compliance auditing can yield many significant findings and recommendations that improve control, reduce costs, and minimize risks. Operations auditing concepts must not be overlooked entirely during even the most restricted of financial audits for they may point to problems of an operations nature rather than mere lapses in internal control and employee compliance.

NOTES

1. Victor Z. Brink and James A. Cashin, *Internal Auditing* (New York: The Ronald Press Company, 1958), pp. 16–18.

2. L. E. Sweeney, "Are Internal Auditors Responsible for Fraud Detection?" *Internal Auditor*, August 1976, p. 12.

3. L. B. Sawyer, "What's the Internal Auditor's Responsibility for Preventing and Detecting Fraud, Grandfather?" *Internal Auditor*, June 1974, p. 79.

4. A. E. Marien, "Internal Auditing and Psychological Patterns," *Hospital Financial Management*, October 1968, pp. 26–27, 29.

5. G. W. Gooche, "Methods and Control of Embezzlement," *Medical Group Management*, January 1970, pp. 11–12.

6. M. J. Barrett and L. R. Radde, "Top Management Fraud: Something Can Be Done Now!" *Internal Auditor*, October 1976, p. 28.

7. B. J. Knamm, "Small Hospitals Can Afford Internal Control," *Hospital Financial Management*, May 1972, pp. 28–30.

8. E. J. Wolff, "Accounting Controls," *Hospital Financial Management*, May 1970, p. 15.

Chapter 14

Internal Auditing Applications for Hospital Programs

Many hospital programs and functions might not be considered at first as likely areas for financial, compliance, and operations auditing. Cost containment, records management, and infection control are examples of operations that can benefit from thorough reviews by internal auditors. The auditors can contribute directly to reducing costs by assisting certified public accountants in their work. The more internal auditors can help CPAs, the better will be the audit coverage and the lower the costs of the CPA engagement. There are other areas in hospitals that at first may not seem susceptible to internal auditing reviews, but many possible applications can be found. Examples of areas not covered here are: construction contracts and the actual construction, volunteer services, religious services provided to patients, motor pools, and all contracts entered into by the hospital. This chapter provides information on which to base designs for audit programs for cost containment, records management, and infection control and offers insights into how internal auditors can save hospitals substantial sums by reducing the expense of CPA engagements.

ASSISTING CERTIFIED PUBLIC ACCOUNTANTS

As mentioned in Chapter 3, internal auditors may reduce the cost of CPA engagements by 10 to 15 percent. It is safe to assume that savings will grow with increases in the quality of hospital internal auditing programs and the degree of independence auditors have. It also may be assumed the overall quality of the CPA audit can be expected to improve because the firm's personnel will be able to concentrate on matters of more importance, leaving much of the routine work to the internal auditors. Finally, internal auditors help reduce CPA fees by perfecting the hospital's internal controls. CPAs can reduce their work in areas where good internal control is demonstrated.[1]

Below are ten sets of checkpoints that can be used to help determine whether internal auditing is making its maximum contribution to reducing CPA costs and to improving overall audit quality, and whether the CPA firm accepts the concept of using the internal auditors to reduce its time on the job.

1. Has there been a sustained effort to coordinate all phases of annual audit programs to provide maximum coverage and to eliminate overlaps? Has the hospital's director participated in planning this coordination?
2. Does a written plan exist for improving the CPA firm's use of internal auditing's work? Does the plan discuss staffing, independence, reporting, and audit coverage as they relate to internal auditing?
3. Does the working relationship between the internal auditing staff and CPA personnel provide for a maximum of sharing of ideas and viewpoints?[2] Does the CPA firm freely share its plans, audit programs, and reports? Some firms may believe too much sharing with internal auditors is not desirable and will compromise their independence. There is evidence to support the view that sharing at this level, which makes maximum use of internal auditing's contribution to reducing fees, does not threaten the independence of outside auditors.[3]
4. Does the CPA firm advise internal auditors on technical matters such as audit program design and improved methods for performing work? Does the CPA firm share computer auditing software packages?
5. Does the CPA firm provide training programs for internal auditors? Internal auditing directors may have difficulty providing adequate staff training on some subjects such as flow charting and analysis, statistical sampling, and computer auditing.
6. Do internal auditors cooperate freely with CPA personnel? Are all internal auditing reports, workpapers, and other pertinent information supplied to the CPA firm? Do internal auditors regularly brief CPA staff in operating changes and provide orientations for new CPA personnel?
7. Does the internal auditing function participate to a maximum extent in the year-end audit? Do internal auditors assist in reviews of cash, confirmation of receivables and payables, and physical inventories in the form of joint audits?
8. Is the internal auditing function safeguarded against compromising its own operations auditing approach? Although internal auditors do perform financial and compliance audits and must assist CPA firms as much as possible, they must not devote too much time to these two areas and cause the hospital to lose most of the benefits of operations auditing reviews.
9. Does the director of internal auditing report to the hospital director any findings as to the adequacy of the CPA firm's work? Does the CPA firm

report to the hospital director the adequacy of the internal auditing function's work?

10. What provision has been made for measuring and reporting the cost effectiveness of increased internal auditing activity in reducing CPA costs and overall coverage? How does this experience compare with other hospitals?

These checkpoints should be covered jointly by the CPA firm's partner in charge, the director of internal auditing, and the hospital administrator. Much is to be gained by improving cooperation between hospital internal auditors and CPA firms. Top management must take a positive interest in the process. While many CPA firms actively support increased use of internal auditors, some may not. Regardless of the exact situation, both the hospital's administration and director of internal auditing must advocate increased cooperation.

EVALUATING COST CONTAINMENT PROGRAMS

The cost of health care has become a national issue as ever greater sums of money are expended by the public. Since the early 1950s the spending has almost doubled as measured as a percentage of the gross national product.[4] Many factors contribute to these increasing costs: higher wages for hospital employees, larger and more sophisticated facilities, insurance reimbursement based on costs, increased services, much higher malpractice insurance, and inflation. National priorities are dictating a shift in perspective from developing and delivering better quality health care to providing it at a reasonable cost with carefully controlled sacrifices of quality.

Internal auditors can play a vital role in containing health care costs in two respects: (1) identifying inefficiencies in hospital operations and (2) evaluating hospital cost containment efforts. Cost containment has proved to be a controversial issue. Many of the factors that most affect costs (number of cases treated, length of stay, case mix, and intensity and scope of service) are not susceptible to control. Further, there is no agreement on what constitutes reasonable quality care. Many costs can be reduced by altering the type of care (professional services and facilities), but, without agreement as to what services are essential, few hospitals will commit themselves voluntarily to a "no frills" program of health care. A last issue is that hospitals traditionally have not had incentives for holding costs down. To date, no programs devised to provide incentives for restraining costs have been found effective.[5]

Because of these three factors, it may be necessary for a regulatory agency such as the government or the Joint Commission on Accreditation of Hospitals to establish external cost controls that hospital administrators will accept more readily.

If a voluntary system of cost controls is to work, hospitals must get on board conceptually with the theme of cost containment and begin establishing operating goals that do restrain expenditures and develop information systems to evaluate quality, cost, and service effectiveness. Incentives can be supplied by the government, the marketplace, and voluntary organizations without imposing operating standards. Examples of these types of incentives are establishing operating standards such as occupancy rates, reducing staffing per patient-day, and developing performance measures that can be compared among hospitals.

Cost containment programs, whether imposed or voluntary, must operate effectively. Internal auditors must assure themselves and the governing board that the hospital's administrators are controlling costs successfully. Effective cost containment programs have a number of attributes that can be evaluated during an operations review. Below are ten sets of checkpoints that should be found in most cost containment programs.

1. Who is responsible for the hospital's cost containment program? Has a committee been formed? If so, what is its composition, its goals, its powers? Are its operating procedures written down?

2. Have clear, attainable, and measurable goals been selected for all hospital areas? Are the goals in agreement with the institution's goals? Do cost containment policies complement overall operating policies?

3. Are the efforts of the cost containment program directed properly? Has the overall direction of the program been to cut costs wherever possible rather than to prepare a process of meaningful cost effectiveness studies leading to well-planned decisions on expenditures?

4. How thorough is the committee's work? Are in-depth cost finding studies made that identify all expenses? Are the costs broken down further on a range from fixed to variable? Are utilization studies performed where necessary?

5. Does top management support the program? What reports and recommendations are received from the cost containment program? What actions result?

6. Does the committee exhibit originality and resourcefulness in dealing with cost containment problems? Does the committee request several alternate proposals for dealing with particular problems of departments so as to be able to make more informed decisions? Creativity and resourcefulness are two attributes essential to the program's success.

7. What specific areas have been reviewed since the program's inception? Have shared services been analyzed to avoid unnecessary duplications among local hospitals? What services are shared: laundry, purchasing, food service, computer, microfilming? Have ambulatory and outpatient services been reviewed for increases in such areas as surgery or hemodi-

alysis? Have staffing levels been analyzed and put under continuing supervision? Are job descriptions, organization charts, and operating statistics requested before approving new positions or refilling existing positions?

8. Have cost containing incentive systems been implemented to encourage all employees to spot potential areas for savings? Are employees motivated to improve their own performances? Are performance incentive systems directed at individuals, teams, and larger groups? What efforts have been made to make physicians more cost conscious?

9. Have advanced financial control systems been implemented and do they effectively identify all costs for all areas? How is this information used by the committee?

10. Has the committee dealt effectively with the more obvious areas where cost savings can be achieved? Has the pharmacy's inventory been examined to reduce inventories, have computer services been examined for improved and reduced utilization, have the cafeteria's costs and revenues been analyzed, and have all opportunities at marketing the hospital's services been explored?

Internal auditors will come upon many aspects of hospital operation that can be referred to the cost containment program. No other employees have a broader and more complete understanding of hospital operations than the internal auditors. This familiarity can be put to use by evaluating the cost containment program's adequacy in terms of how thoroughly it covers each area and the hospital as a whole.

EVALUATING THE RECORDS MANAGEMENT PROGRAM

The need for good records has been increasing steadily. The absence of good patient care and business records can have costly consequences—for example, repayments to Medicare for undocumented charges, and loss of charges and collections in the business system. The management of medical records has been recognized as a profession with special education and certification programs. Records management in general also has been recognized formally as an important aspect of all organizations, large or small. No hospital can afford to be without a sound records management program that provides clear guidelines for what types of information must be kept and where, with what security and safeguards, and for how long. Internal auditors must review the various systems and procedures that compose the records management programs for hospital medical and business areas. Below are ten sets of checkpoints on which to begin an audit program design.

1. Do all records have definite retention and destruction schedules? Who developed the policies and were they approved by the governing board?

Is there a continuing program of records management, with personnel assigned to carry it out?

2. Do retention schedules meet applicable federal and state regulations? Do the schedules meet the hospital's needs for records while not keeping an excessive volume of material on hand?

3. Has adequate consideration been given to the types of records and their retention schedules? The issue here is one of economics. A policy may require records to be retained for a specific period to document a transaction with a patient or employee. Experience may indicate the records seldom are used after a year and that the risk of loss from disposing of them is less than the cost of storing them. The auditor should recommend the retention schedule be reexamined and adjusted to bring the storage costs more in line with the risks involved.

4. Are there enough types of records? Are they organized in such a way as to minimize paper processing needs and provide maximum documentation and information? Is there much duplication of records in part or in full? Do departments routinely retain documentation of charges that also are kept by the business office?

5. Are the records retained in a manner that facilitates quick retrieval and accurate filing? There are many proved methods for organizing all types of records, including using various types of equipment. Auditors must be alert for requests for records that require an extended amount of work to locate.

6. What use is made of a central records storage facility? Is it properly equipped and staffed? Is its service well known throughout the hospital? Is it properly utilized?

7. What use has been made of microfilm in the business record area? If data processing is used, for business purposes, have applications of computer output microfilm been explored?

8. How are important records safeguarded from loss or destruction? Are storage areas clean and well organized? Are the policies and procedures for record access and removal adequate and are they followed?

9. How are records destroyed? Do the hospital's procedures for disposing of records and trash ensure maximum confidentiality?

10. Is the generating of new reports and forms monitored by an administrator? Is the staff generally informed of what records are available? Is there an index of all of the hospital's records?

Hospitals must have an effective program of records management to meet federal and state regulations, the needs of documentation for substantiating transactions with patients and employees, and their own needs to operate. Internal auditors can make an excellent contribution to records management by reviewing the program in total and then checking out its performance at each location audited. Since internal auditors are dependent on good records for audit trails, there seldom is a better scrutiny of records than theirs.

EVALUATING INFECTION CONTROL PROGRAMS

An operations audit of a program such as hospital-wide infection control is a unique undertaking for internal auditors. Effective infection control programs have as their goal reducing the number of infections patients acquire while in the hospital and minimizing the spread of infection to the community. Although internal auditors cannot deal with the medical aspects of infection control, they certainly can perform operations evaluations of the administrative aspects. A recent review of the literature on the subject yielded a substantial number of administrative points that may be incorporated in an audit program. The following ten sets of checkpoints cover most such aspects.

1. What are the goals of the hospital's infection control program? What precautions are taken for preventing harm to patients? Does the infection control program also include employees, visitors, and the community?
2. What objectives have been established? Do they include the means for data gathering on the incidence of infection, effective reporting of infection occurrence ratios that are higher than normal, remedial and preventive actions, review and evaluation of antibiotic usages, and education?
3. Has an infection control committee been formed? Is it chaired by the hospital epidemiologist? Does it have a heterogenous membership including infection control officers and representatives of nursing, pharmacy, microbiology, surgery, housekeeping, dietary, and the emergency room?
4. Has the committee carefully documented the methodology to be used to monitor infections? This is essential not only for purposes of management but also for the scientific aspects of infection control that require data to be gathered in the same consistent method over long periods. In particular, have the methods for reviewing infection reports, for inspecting equipment, for reporting, and for recordkeeping been established clearly?
5. Is there an effective program of infection control education? Does it cover all pertinent areas and employees?
6. To what extent do physicians and nurses cooperate by reporting infections? Are infections reported only on a cyclical basis after periodic pressures are brought by the infection control committee? Lack of cooperation will result in unreliable data.
7. Does the hospital employ a full-time or part-time infection control nurse? The position generally is regarded as full-time for hospitals of 400 beds

or more. Infection control nurses often are made necessary because of noncooperation by physicians and nurses.

8. How are the data processed and reported? Is electronic data processing available?
9. What documentation is maintained on corrective actions by physicians and departments? When it is necessary to confront a physician or department on poor health care practices, is the action documented carefully to ensure that an accurate record is created for future reference? When corrective action is necessary, are the positive educational aspects, rather than the punitive aspects, stressed?
10. How does the hospital compare with national averages? What legal actions are pending on infections acquired while in the hospital?

It is obvious internal auditors can make operations evaluations of hospital infection control programs. However, they should not stop here. This is but one example of a program that at first would appear completely beyond the scope of internal auditing. Hospitals have a broad assortment of programs, all of which should be analyzed for possible applications of operations auditing. Many of these programs can benefit from an operations review.

CONCLUSION

Internal auditors must be alert for possible applications of financial, compliance, and operations auditing in hospitals. Every activity, department, and program should be identified and examined for possible internal audit reviews. There will be few instances in which a well-informed auditor cannot make some contribution. Even where most of the issue is medical or technical, there usually can be found an underlying administrative structure that can benefit from a thorough internal audit review.

SUMMARY OF PART IV

The last five chapters have provided numerous practical applications for internal auditing in hospitals. Internal auditors will be challenged continually to provide comprehensive, thorough, and professional coverage. It has been emphasized repeatedly that auditors must prepare themselves for each audit by reviewing literature on the function to be reviewed. The audit checklists provided here form only a basic framework on which to build thorough audit programs. While many of the checkpoints can be used in many other projects, in the end it is the responsibility of the internal auditor writing the audit program to prepare one uniquely fitted to the particular hospital and function. This will require a solid knowledge of the subject that can be gained only by thorough preliminary research.

Part V will take up with practical applications for internal auditing in teaching hospitals. Teaching hospitals often are larger and more complex than most others and require that special attention be directed to their internal auditing needs.

NOTES

1. W. B. Haase, "Cooperation Makes the Difference," *Internal Auditor*, August 1973, p. 45.

2. Ibid., p. 42.

3. Victor Z. Brink, James A. Cashin, and Herbert Witt, *Modern Internal Auditing: An Operational Approach* (New York: The Ronald Press Company, 1973), p. 680.

4. Rockwell Schulz and Alton C. Johnson, *Management of Hospitals* (New York: McGraw-Hill Book Company, 1976), p. 203.

5. Ibid., p. 215.

Internal Auditing in Academic Medical Centers

Chapter 15

Evaluating the Academic Medical Center's Organization and Leadership

Part V continues the discussion of practical applications of internal auditing by introducing the most complicated organizational environment in which hospital internal auditors will have to work: the university medical center. Academic medical centers are composed of a medical school and possibly others such as dentistry and pharmacy, and a hospital that usually is administered separately. The size, number, and importance of academic medical centers has increased dramatically since World War II when the federal government became a sponsor of improved medical education and research.

Today the need for sound administrative organization and leadership has become crucial to the continuing well-being of academic medical centers. Medical center administrators must oversee research, teaching, and patient care activities in a managerial environment filled with the influences of departments, faculty, chairpeople, committees, students, employees, campus interests, community interests, state and federal legislation, granting agencies, and the Veterans Hospital administrative system.

Efforts to evaluate administrative, organizational, and leadership needs of academic medical centers have identified many of the principle issues that confront their administrators, but have not found solutions to the problems these issues pose. Internal auditors will find many opportunities for assisting the medical centers in coping more effectively with complexities and influences that make effective administration difficult. Many of the major areas of concern presented here will be encountered as internal auditors work their way through the centers' departments and programs. The detailed experience of management's successes and failures that auditors acquire in projects at the department level will prepare them to contribute to the solution of many major administrative problems. Regardless of the complexities, it is possible to develop successful administration based on clearly established goals and objectives, written policies and procedures, and sound organization.

RELATIONS WITH UNIVERSITY ADMINISTRATION

There are many diverse approaches for integrating academic medical centers with university campuses. This is the result of a number of factors that must be taken into consideration when dealing with medical centers and their integration and autonomy. First, academic medical centers often are the second largest academic units on campus, behind the faculty of arts and science. They often require the largest fiscal resources and physical facilities. Second, the centers have important community links as a result of their health care services. In addition, the teaching physicians who constitute the clinical faculty play important roles in medical centers and, because of their patient care activities, differ from fellow faculty members such as those in law and engineering who do not have direct community impact. And, third, university administrations may not be fully staffed and prepared to meet the rigors of managing what have become extremely large campuses.

These factors plus others unique to each campus and academic medical center cause the issues of integration and autonomy to be resolved in many different ways, each custom fitted to the particular administrative situations encountered. Internal auditors should explore the nature of the integration and autonomy to ensure the relationship has been well-planned and well-documented and in fact contributes to achieving campus and medical center goals. The checkpoints below are starting points for further thought.

1. Who is the highest administrative official of the medical center and to what position does that person report? The position preferably should report to the president of the university or to the chancellor if the medical school is a member of a campus that in turn is only one of a number of campuses.[1] In most instances the medical school and hospital will have entirely separate line organizations, in which case the heads of the medical school and the hospital both should report to the campus official. The auditor must be certain the position reported to does represent the campus as a whole and not merely a segment of it.

2. If the academic medical center also includes other schools such as dentistry, pharmacy, public health, and allied health sciences, the top administrator should not also be the director of one of the schools. The top administrator must be in a position to render fair, objective decisions and not have them impeached because of possible favoritism toward one or another organizational component.

3. The Commission for the Study of the Governance of the Academic Medical Center recommended medical schools be integrated fully with university campuses and follow campus academic and fiscal policies and procedures.[2] Internal auditors must verify the extent to which this is accomplished while

also being alert for instances where exceptions to campus policies and procedures should be granted. Academic promotions and tenure decisions must be designed to deal specifically with the patient care aspect of the medical school. While medical schools should be integrated with university campuses, hospitals affiliated with academic medical centers frequently are and probably should be autonomous from the campus. Hospitals have demonstrable administrative needs that require freedom from campus policies and procedures. Fiscal exceptions are necessary to deal with needs of the hospital's patient care activities. Exceptions also may be needed in purchasing, salary administration, budgeting, and finance.

4. Medical schools must have written goals, objectives, policies, and procedures available for review. Who created them and who approved them? Are they complete and up to date? Are they compatible with those of the campus? Other schools of the medical center should be reviewed.

5. Is the medical school's administration organized and staffed properly? Is there an organization chart? Are there position descriptions? What has been employee turnover for these positions? Lack of continuity in leadership can have drastic consequences for medical centers. Other schools also must.be reviewed.

Internal auditors should find a clear, well-designed pattern for conducting academic and fiscal business between medical centers and university campuses. If they are missing, the auditor should advocate the relationships be planned and documented to improve administrative control and understanding.

LEADERSHIP OF MEDICAL SCHOOLS

It is generally agreed the dean must be the locus for leadership and must be capable of coordinating and balancing the many conflicting forces within the medical school and the medical center. The importance of the dean's administrative role has increased significantly in the last 20 years as the size and complexity of medical schools and centers has grown. As the new demands of greater size, greater amounts of research, and better fiscal management have arisen, there has been increased turnover among deans that has undermined the continuity of leadership seriously. The increased turnover rate can be attributed to the considerable pressures of the job that often have been aggravated by the existence of many avoidable administrative problems. Internal auditors will not be able to reduce the pressures deans experience but certainly may help them by spotting operating problems that contribute unnecessarily to their difficulties. Following are five areas internal auditors should explore to ensure the dean is provided with every opportunity to lead the medical center in a successful pursuit of its goals.

1. Is the dean's position described accurately and are the powers of the position sufficient to meet the demands made on it? Are organizational and authority relationships between the dean and the many other organizational elements documented? How is the dean expected to relate to various committees, faculty, chairpersons, students, and the hospital's administrator?
2. What types and amounts of support does the dean receive from the campus? Does the campus support the dean solidly or does it meddle constantly in medical center affairs?
3. Does the dean have a staff adequate in numbers and types?[3] Do their organizational relationships promote effective administration?
4. What is the makeup of the remainder of the medical school's organization? Do many of the departments resemble empires, do they lack professional administration, and do they invariably pursue their own goals to the exclusion of the medical school's?
5. Does the medical center have adequate communications? How are faculty and employees kept informed of the many changes that occur constantly? In particular, what types of publications are generated and how are they distributed? Is there a lack of coordination among the publications? Can they be combined or some eliminated?

Internal auditors must review Chapter 10 (Evaluating Top Management Performance) for its many possible applications here. It is important to note the dean's job is exceedingly difficult even with good overall organization and administration. With anything less, the dean will be required to expend much energy and time constantly fighting fires, with little time left to tackle the harder problems that produce the fires.

Internal auditors must be patient when advocating change. While the wisdom of a change may be accepted, implementing it can take months or even years. This is the result of the large size of academic medical centers, the many negotiations required with the numerous special interests involved, and the limited amount of time the dean can contribute to solving the problems.

DEPARTMENT HEADS AND FACULTY ADMINISTRATIVE ROLES

Medical schools are composed of departments that specialize in various basic sciences such as anatomy and physiology and in clinical areas such as surgery and internal medicine.[4] The responsibilities of these two types of departments vary. Basic science departments educate medical students, as do clinical departments, but the latter also must train interns, residents, and postdoctoral fellows. All departments are led by chairpersons who are responsible for teaching, patient care, research, and administration in their areas. Faculty members generally are provided an opportunity to serve on one or more medical school or hospital committees. This achieves a broad base of faculty support and responsibility for medical center affairs. Internal auditors should determine whether the existing organization and policies provide for sound departmental management and a broad base of faculty participation.

1. What are the medical school's recruiting methods and selection criteria for department heads? Recruiting has become progressively more difficult as chair positions become less attractive and the pool of qualified applicants shrinks. These problems are caused in part by decreased federal government support of research. The ideal chairperson will have a strong research background and will continue in that work after appointment to help lead the department in pursuit of project funding—one criterion for getting the job. However, with fewer grant dollars available, department heads find it harder to lead that research thrust and, as dollars dwindle, so, too, does the number of individuals performing research. Other important attributes for department heads are experience in teaching and demonstrated leadership and administrative skills. For clinical departments, the chairperson also must be an excellent physician.

2. Are department heads appointed for fixed periods with the opportunity for reappointment? A minimum of five years is recommended to ensure continuity of leadership, which is especially important in clinical departments. Rotating leaders is not recommended.[5] Does the dean actively evaluate their performance and, where needed, remove those who fail to lead their departments effectively?

3. Are the departments organized along medical subspecialties? Is there a proliferation of departments that results in confusion? It is recommended that subspecialties, especially within major departments, remain within those units as divisions with their own leadership that reports to the chair.

4. Has the dean established goals, objectives, and standards of performance for academic departments and are the heads aware of them and support them? Are the goals and objectives realistic and measurable? Are the standards of performance clear and, if met, will they fulfill the goals?

5. Has adequate attention been provided to organizing committees for the participation of department heads and faculty in the governance of the medical center? Are the chairs formed into an advisory committee to the dean? Are there faculty committees that control admissions, curriculum, student affairs, faculty appointments? What committees exist for faculty participation in the running of the hospital? Does the faculty appear to have a broad participation in the operation of the medical center?

Internal auditors should expect to find most of these points in every medical center. The absence of any of them should be questioned. There will be a wide variation in how each medical school achieves its organization of departments, selects and retains its chairpersons, and acquires a broad base of faculty support and responsibility in governance. Thoughtful inquiries by the auditor may lead to reflective thinking on the part of the dean, department heads, and faculty members as to how the existing arrangements could be improved.

CONCLUSION

Academic medical centers have proved to be very resistant to vigorous administration and perhaps are not subject to as rigorous controls as hospitals alone. Internal auditors can play vital a role in appraising medical center administration and leadership by surfacing problem areas and issues that have not been dealt with effectively but that detract from the center's operating atmosphere. In many instances, the auditor will be able to recommend to the dean only a possible course of action to be evaluated. Regardless of the difficulties of finding sound answers to problems and overcoming the many delays involved in implementing changes, internal auditors always must advocate effective leadership, sound organization, and written policies and procedures and assure themselves the management processes of planning, staffing, directing, and controlling are occurring.

NOTES

1. O. C. Elder, Jr., "The 1980 University Medical Center: Its Mission and Administration," *Journal of Medical Education*, March 1973, p. 229.

2. *Report of the Commission for the Study of the Governance of the Academic Medical Center* (New York: Josiah Macy, Jr. Foundation, 1970), p. 19.

3. J. W. Fredrickson, "Organizing for Better Medical School Management," *Hospital Care Management Review*, Spring 1977, pp. 72–73.

4. P. R. Lee, "A Tiger By the Tail: The Governance of the Academic Health Sciences Center," *Journal of Medical Education*, January 1973, p. 32.

5. Macy Report, op. cit., p. 38.

Auditing Medical School Management

Medical schools and large hospitals have many of the same management needs. Medical schools have large sums of funds to budget and control; however, the types of funds involved produce unique management problems. Most medical schools are supported by a combination of state appropriations, gifts and endowments, and professional fee income. They have large and varied personnel, administration, and payroll control needs. Unique to their environment are academic appointments, staff paid from research grants that may be lost, and problems of equitably distributing professional fee income earned by the teaching physicians. Medical schools also control equipment and supply inventories. Their needs differ from those of hospitals, however, in that much of the equipment in research laboratories may have been purchased with federal grants that restrict ownership and portability. There are many other areas of similarities. These examples provide an ample basis for discussing internal auditing applications and, in fact, cover the major topics of medical school management.

FUND MANAGEMENT, BUDGETING, AND ACCOUNTING CONTROL

Medical schools receive funds from a variety of sources, with the degree of support from each source varying widely. To gain optimum use of these funds, sound budgeting practices must be combined with accurate and timely accounting control and reporting. A key difference between a successful medical school and academic department and the average medical school or department hinges on how well each performs its budgeting and accounting functions. Internal auditors can make many contributions toward perfecting those practices, based in part on the ten sets of checkpoints below.

1. Does the medical school have short-range and long-range plans and accompanying budgets? Are they realistic? What budgeting and reporting

mechanisms are used to control budgets? Do departments have all of the above?

2. Is the annual budget process well-planned and well-coordinated? Is sufficient time provided? Is there adequate documentation to support decision making and the actual budgeting process?

3. Does the medical school examine department budgets to ensure the budgeting process has been carried out intelligently and provides for maximum utilization of resources? Internal auditors should review Chapter 10 for other budgeting checkpoints.

4. What type of accounting system is used to control expenditures? Is there a central accounting office or do the various departments do their own accounting? Do departments have uniform accounting systems and do they work? What use could be made of a computer at either the central or departmental level?

5. What role does the campus have in fund accounting? Are campus policies and procedures followed? What computing support does the campus supply? Is it accurate and timely?

6. What has been the medical school's experience with past audits of federal grants? Have all audit criticisms been dealt with? Have expenditures been disallowed and repaid by the medical school? What procedures are enforced to ensure that expenditures of funds comply with the requirements of granting agencies?

7. Who prepares federal reports on expenditures? Based on what information? Are reports that affect departments and the medical school routinely distributed to them?

8. How successful has the accounting system been in controlling the funds? Have grants expired with unused funds remaining? Have grants been overused seriously, requiring sudden shifts of expenditures to other funding sources?

9. Are all transactions supervised and documented adequately? Is documentation retained long enough to meet federal audit requirements?

10. Are the budgeting and accounting processes staffed and equipped adequately? Are they accomplished at a justifiable cost?

Internal auditors will find many other important checkpoints to consider when evaluating medical school and departmental budgeting and accounting. Many of the chapters in Part IV have checkpoints that can be applied here.

PERSONNEL AND PAYROLL ADMINISTRATION

Proper handling of medical school personnel is challenging because of the wide assortment of positions needed. Medical schools are responsible for handling the personnel and payroll affairs of highly skilled and highly paid physicians, teaching staff, and administrators, as well as file clerks and janitors. Medical schools must be prepared to handle these responsibilities as well as to provide an equitable salary and wage structure.

1. Are all nonacademic positions described properly? Have they been compared with one another to ensure equal pay for equal work? Who is responsible for managing the numbers and types of positions? Do all departments use the same criteria in describing positions and for establishing salary ranges?

2. Do department heads use reasonably comparable methods for deciding at what levels to appoint new faculty? Do they have acceptable methods for deciding on promotion and tenure? The reader should review the personnel administration section in Chapter 12 for more audit checkpoints.

3. What written policies and procedures exist for payroll and personnel? Are they complete and in compliance with all federal and state laws? Are they in agreement with university policies and procedures?

4. Are the departments adequately staffed to handle payroll and personnel matters? Are the employees responsible properly trained? Do the departments have procedures for handling related areas such as interviewing, orientation, evaluation, and training? Is there a central personnel office for the medical school, and is it properly staffed? What authority and powers do the departments have?

5. What use is made of centralized processing of more routine activities, such as personnel records and payroll? Are electronic data processing applications adequate?

6. Are there written procedures that cover payroll? Is the system used the same as the campus's or is it one specifically designed for the medical school's needs? When applicable, how is salary that is paid directly to physicians from off-campus sources, such as other hospitals or the Veterans Administration, accounted for? The reader should review the payroll section of Chapter 13 for additional audit checkpoints.

7. Are the departments responsible for all payroll-related records such as vacation, sick leave, and time reports? Are the departments visited periodically by personnel of the medical school or campus central payroll office to audit payroll records?

8. Is there a uniform system of processing time sheets, absences, and payroll among departments? If not, does each department have a system that effectively controls payroll in terms of accuracy and timeliness? Do some departments generate numerous problems and complaints about payroll matters?

MEDICAL CENTER INVENTORIES

Unlike hospitals, medical centers purchase much less equipment and fewer supplies, primarily because administrative, teaching, and research needs do not require investment in the vast array of expensive equipment and supplies that patient care, surgical, and diagnostic areas need. Research requiring highly expensive equipment in the teaching hospital often will have funds from the institution or grants to pay for the use of hospital equipment rather than for its purchase. Teaching needs require investment in equipment such as microscopes and supplies for the basic sciences. While medical centers have less equipment and fewer supplies than hospitals, the difference is only relative because the size and value of the center's materials is quite large. Internal auditors should be certain all of the medical school's inventories are managed properly.

1. Are supplies for teaching areas centrally stocked and controlled? Who is responsible for the management of the supplies? Do the teaching areas and storage rooms appear to be stocked adequately, and are they orderly and clean?

2. Are all purchases for research laboratories handled centrally or by each lab? How are flammable and corrosive supplies stored? If there are hospital storerooms for common supplies, do research laboratories have access?

3. Is there a central supply room for office supplies? Is there a proliferation of types of office supplies? Do offices routinely order from local companies at a cost higher than the central storeroom's?

4. What effort is made to coordinate supply ordering and storage with the hospital? Are larger quantity discounts available? What supplies are available from the campus supply rooms?

5. Is there an accurate record of all equipment in the medical school? What is the dollar value of the materiality level for accounting for equipment? Is it reasonable? Are equipment purchases supported by grant funding screened to avoid unnecessary duplications?

6. What procedures exist for managing warranties and maintenance agreements? Are warranties controlled carefully by various laboratories, offices, and departments? Are maintenance agreements monitored so as to include maximum numbers of pieces of equipment to achieve quantity discounts?

7. Are records maintained to show the source of funds used to purchase equipment, the date of purchase, serial numbers, inventory numbers, location, and state of repair? Does the dean support a policy of interlaboratory and interdepartmental sharing of equipment? Are there core areas

where large, expensive pieces of equipment are housed and operated by trained technicians for all labs?

8. What efforts have been made to develop information and expertise in selecting equipment? Are there specific recommendations on the types of typewriters, word processing equipment, and research laboratory equipment?

9. How often are equipment and supply inventories counted? Who does the counting and reporting? The reader should review Chapter 13 for more audit checkpoints on inventories of supplies and equipment.

10. Is equipment shared by the hospital and the medical school monitored carefully so as to permit equitable distribution of operating costs? Does the hospital claim depreciation on shared equipment?

Inventories of supplies and equipment must be managed and accounted for properly to ensure that medical schools achieve optimum use of their resources and prevent unnecessary assumptions of risks. Internal auditors should call on their experience from auditing the hospital to spot possible improvements and instances where the hospital, teaching areas, and research laboratories can share storage areas and common supply sources for larger quantity discounts.

CONCLUSIONS

Academic medical centers have many important management needs that often are more difficult to fulfill than those in large hospitals. Failure to accomplish effective management will produce immediate wastes of resources and lower overall performance by all areas of the medical center. Internal auditors can make valuable contributions to academic medical centers.

SUMMARY OF PART V

Chapter 16 concludes the discussion of practical applications of internal auditing in the health care and teaching environment. There are countless applications of internal auditing. Internal auditors will be challenged to find and apply these applications to individual projects and to the overall hospital and medical center audit program.

Part VI

Evaluating Internal Auditing's Effectiveness and Future Applications

Chapter 17

Internal Auditing's Contribution to Hospitals

Internal auditing must compete for hospital resources. Top management must be able to measure the function's contribution to hospital goals to determine the resources to allocate to internal auditing and to decide whether it is earning its way. The dilemma faced by top management and directors of internal auditing is how to measure performance.

There are three fundamental measurement problems:

1. Operations auditing usually produces qualitative results that require the efforts of others to implement and have benefits that extend over a considerable operating area or period of time.
2. The better internal auditing performs, the fewer will be the contributions it can make eventually. It may approach a maintenance level requiring a continuing program of internal audits just as before, but the results of many of the projects merely will confirm that the operating status of audited departments still meets the hospital director's standards.
3. Internal auditing is an active ingredient of a hospital's overall system of internal controls. Auditing acts as a surveilling force for top management that ensures all internal controls are sound and are being complied with by employees.

The issue of measuring internal auditing's performance and its contribution to hospital operations should be dealt with in three ways. First, the director of internal auditing must have a program for evaluating the performance of individual auditors and the value of their report findings and recommendations. Second, top management must find acceptable qualitative and quantitative measures of performance. The director of internal auditing also should try to provide some measurements for management's consideration. Third, the use of an external evaluator—either the hospital's CPA firm or a consultant—can be a useful method of measurement.

SELF-EVALUATION BY INTERNAL AUDITING

A soundly conceived program of self-evaluation managed by the director is essential to all internal auditing programs. The degree of formality of the system should fit staff size. In most hospitals, the internal auditing staff usually will have one to five members, including the director. A staff that small requires much personal contact between the director and the other members; as a result, the director will be well informed of each auditor's performance. However, the personal nature of the supervision should not prevent a formal process of evaluation from taking place.

It is recommended the director of internal auditing provide auditors an evaluation after the completion of each program. This is valuable because it provides immediate feedback on individual performance as well as opportunities for improved communication, training, and counseling.[1] If an auditor has performed poorly, the problems causing that result can be pinpointed and discussed while they are fresh on everyone's mind. It may be apparent the person involved requires special training or the director may uncover a poor attitude, poor work habits, or extenuating personal problems.

The evaluation also promotes clear communication between the director and staff members. The employee may wish to point out problems in the administration of the auditing function or encountered on the job. The director will have the opportunity to motivate staff members to continue improvement and encourage them to return to discuss performance problems that they have uncovered on their own.

It is recommended that the director write up the results of the evaluation session. The major findings should be discussed briefly, along with corrective actions to be taken. Although not required, it is preferred that the auditor involved receive a copy. As the number of projects and evaluations increases, the auditor should be demonstrating improvement, documented by better evaluations. If in the end the auditor fails to meet performance standards, the written summaries will make a decision to terminate the individual's employment clear and, in the event of some form of grievance action, should support the termination decision.

The actual evaluation process should have a specific organization that will promote comparison between individual performances and among staff members. Below are general guidelines for producing a performance evaluation format.

1. The auditor's name, the date, the assignment description (including anyone supervised), the number of days and hours budgeted, the actual time required, and the degree of difficulty of the audit must be stated.
2. Performance should be rated on the following points: knowledge, creativity and resourcefulness, speed and accuracy, judgment, ability to follow audit

program instructions, ability to organize and control work, orderliness and neatness of workpapers, written and spoken communication skills, general business consciousness, and ability to work with others.[2]

3. Specific problems and personal weaknesses that affected performance should be identified and the director and auditor should agree on actions to correct the problems and weaknesses.

Internal auditing directors are encouraged to include at least these points in the design of a performance evaluation program. Exactly how this is done or what else is to be included must be left to the discretion of each director.

A second valuable evaluation method is the departmental self-audit. An auditor is assigned this responsibility by the hospital director.[3] Often a newly hired internal auditor with suitable previous experience can perform this duty while maintaining objectivity.[4] The audit program will cover many of the topics presented in Chapters 1 through 9. The auditor will find considerable assistance in designing the self-audit program from available literature. The results of the audit should be presented to the hospital director and director of internal auditing in writing, and corrective action taken as needed. The results of the self-audit also will be of interest to the public accounting firm.

TOP MANAGEMENT'S EVALUATION

The evaluation of internal auditing by top management requires that some form of measurement be adopted. General management experience indicates one of the best methods of ensuring good performance is to have a director of internal auditing who sets high personal standards and whose work ethic corresponds to that of management. Such a director can be expected to press internal auditing staff members toward better performance and to improve on the function's impact on hospital operations. Beyond this guide, efforts at performance measurement must be relied on. A number of general measurement guidelines are presented below.

1. Instances where fraud is uncovered produce immediate and calculable savings for hospitals, not including possible restitution from the employee or employees involved. Top management should require a complete investigation of middle management's failure to control the area involved, including an analysis of the internal controls used by the unit and a review of the internal auditing program that may have failed to spot the fraud. That last factor may have the negative impact of pointing out internal auditing deficiencies.

2. The discovery of obvious wastes and inefficiencies often can produce considerable savings and improvements that are calculable. While the merits of each finding and the need to share the responsibility for the improvement

with the unit's management will vary, some form of equitable dollar figure usually can be calculated as representing internal auditing's contribution. The director of internal auditing may want to note in audit reports the estimated value of the change to document the contribution.

3. The number of times a hospital or teaching medical center is penalized for failure to comply with federal, state, and local laws and with rulings of regulatory agencies and commissions may produce valid measures of internal auditing's performance. Federal audits of grants, contracts, and Medicare can produce exceptionally heavy financial burdens for the hospital or medical center involved. An effective internal auditing program can produce control systems and procedures that ensure compliance with all laws and regulations affecting health care delivery, teaching, and research.

4. Closely related to uncovering waste and inefficiencies is the discovery of missed opportunities to add new services or to change existing ones that will increase revenues. Missed improvement opportunities have a real cost, although they do not show up directly in income calculations. An example might be the ownership of unused land that could be converted to a pay parking lot or leased for some other purpose. Again, the value of the finding can be calculated.

5. Instances of internal auditing interaction with top management can produce valuable performance indicators for evaluation. Top management will be able to assess for itself the overall quality, scope, and timeliness of internal auditing's reporting. Management will be able to judge the soundness of the findings and recommendations and the degree the heads of the audited departments have accepted the work of internal auditing.

6. A last area with calculable savings is the degree by which internal auditing reduces the cost of CPA engagements or improves their effectiveness.

Top management and the director of internal auditing will find performance evaluation of the function a challenge that must be met. All of the above points must be considered in any evaluation scheme. As mentioned before, internal auditing also has a valid role as a part of hospital internal control systems with a cost that must be viewed as the same as those of the accounting department. The evaluation must be made even though no specific guidelines exist for its accomplishment. Resourceful hospital administrators and directors of internal auditing will find many different approaches for accomplishing the evaluation process.

EXTERNAL EVALUATION

External evaluations of internal auditing's performance can be of value if performed on a regular basis by public accountants or on an irregular or crisis basis by special consultants. The CPA firms engaged by hospitals are in the unique position of observing the results of the function's efforts in internal control and in assisting the firms' personnel in their annual audits. [5] It is recommended that hospitals request their CPA firms to evaluate the adequacy of the overall audit program along with recommendations for improvements. However, hospital directors should be alert to instances where the CPA firm takes a narrow approach to the evaluation process by concentrating on financial and internal control matters. The directors also should be aware the CPA firm may concentrate the evaluation on ways the internal auditors can assist the firm's personnel and slight its evaluation of the entire audit program, including operations audits, staffing, training, and quality of work.

Hospitals establishing an internal auditing capability or with operating problems within that function may want to employ an outside consultant. Most management consulting firms have the capability of evaluating the situation and making recommendations to help internal auditing become a solid performer for the hospital.

CONCLUSION

Performance evaluations are a crucial aspect of management that must be carried out in spite of the difficulties of actually measuring work. A sound program of all three forms of evaluation is needed to make possible informed decision making by top management and the director of internal auditing. Internal auditing is a function that can benefit hospitals greatly if it is supported adequately and pressed for maximum performance. Performance evaluation is a key component for allocating hospital resources for internal auditing and for ensuring that the function is yielding its total benefits for the institution's operations.

NOTES

1. P. V. De Lomba, "Measuring the Auditor's Performance," *Internal Auditor*, June 1974, p. 27.
2. Ibid., p. 32.
3. Victor Z. Brink, James A. Cashin, and Herbert Witt, *Modern Internal Auditing: An Operational Approach*. (New York: The Ronald Press Company, 1973), pp. 714–722.
4. E. L. McKinley, "Auditing the Internal Audit Function," *Internal Auditor*, October 1974, p. 53.
5. Ibid., p. 53.

Chapter 18

The Future of Hospital Internal Auditing

The primary purpose of this book has been to advocate the use of internal auditing in hospitals by demonstrating the many benefits this capability can provide. A synthesis of available literature on the subject has been provided and applied to hospitals to educate top managements on the value of the function and how it must work. The key to the future for internal auditing in hospitals and teaching medical centers is the recognition of the function's value by governing boards and hospital directors.

Top managements that give internal auditing the opportunity to prove itself will not be disappointed with the results. During a time when social forces are being concentrated on the nation's health care resources, what better time is there for hospital managements to turn to a function that is dedicated to the same goals as those of society? Regardless of whether integrated health care systems or autonomous hospitals are to manage the health care industry's resources, individual institutions must seek systematically to improve their operations. Internal auditing can be invaluable in achieving this goal.

LOOKING BACK

During the last 30 years, internal auditing has evolved from a role as an internal control and checking function using financial and compliance auditing to one using operations and management auditing to appraise all aspects of an organization. Internal auditing's goals have changed from safeguarding assets to ensuring that operations are efficient and meet standards set by top management. As a profession, internal auditing has grown substantially and now has achieved the formal status of a profession, with a professional organization and journal, professional certification, accepted standards of performance, a code of ethics, and a common body of knowledge. The organizational status of internal auditing has improved considerably to the point where it is recognized as a valuable function that should report directly to the board of directors. Internal auditing has come a long way, indeed.

LOOKING AHEAD

Internal auditing is still evolving and there are many goals left to accomplish. Its role continues to broaden to include all operations and all levels of management. It is becoming an important ingredient for appraising the adequacy and representativeness of management information systems. Management auditing responsibilities will include ever greater levels of appraisal of planning, organizing, staffing, directing, and controlling by all executive levels. Ultimately, the internal auditor must determine whether the organization's various programs and departments are working together harmoniously toward the institution's overall goals. Internal auditing's goals may even reach out to encompass concepts of social responsibility and environmental impact.

The profession should continue to grow as larger numbers of internal auditors are employed by all industries. Demands will be made on the profession to improve auditing techniques and develop new types of audit programs covering an ever larger number of organizational functions. Increased recognition of internal auditing must be emphasized on college and university campuses until it becomes standard course material. The organizational status of the function can be expected to improve as more organizations acquire an internal auditing capability and as more auditors report directly to the board of directors.

THE DAWN OF HOSPITAL INTERNAL AUDITING

A survey of 350 hospitals recently completed by the author indicated 15 percent of those responding had what they considered to be active internal auditing capabilities and 9 percent more were planning on adding the capability in the near future. The remaining 76 percent did not perceive a need for an internal auditing capability. The hospitals reporting they were using the function usually employed one auditor and on the average had had internal auditing for only four years. These findings provide considerable room for improved utilization of internal auditing by the health care industry and provide a new frontier for practitioners to explore. The Institute of Internal Auditors has begun a program of seminars for hospital internal auditors and more literature is becoming available.

For internal auditing to enjoy the full light of day in the health care industry, much more needs to be accomplished. Hospital management associations and organizations must be convinced to support the function. Hospital administrators and boards of directors must be educated about internal auditing and encouraged to give it a try. Members of local Institute of Internal Auditor chapters should take it upon themselves to gain their support for improved hospital operating efficiency through the use of their expertise.

More research is needed to determine optimal hospital internal auditing staff sizes and composition, organization status, and types of personnel to recruit. Expanded training opportunities must be provided by professional organizations and colleges and universities.

Hospital internal auditing is in its ascendency and must rise to take its place in the management of the health care industry. The diligent efforts of many persons will be required to accomplish this. Advocates of internal auditing can rest assured it is a valuable function that can provide affective services to hospitals and, indirectly, to the local community and the entire industry.

Standards for the Professional Practice of Internal Auditing

Introduction

Internal auditing is an independent appraisal function established within an organization to examine and evaluate its activities as a service to the organization. The objective of internal auditing is to assist members of the organization in the effective discharge of their responsibilities. To this end, internal auditing furnishes them with analyses, appraisals, recommendations, counsel, and information concerning the activities reviewed.

The members of the organization assisted by internal auditing include those in management and the board of directors. Internal auditors owe a responsibility to both, providing them with information about the adequacy and effectiveness of the organization's system of internal control and the quality of performance. The information furnished to each may differ in format and detail, depending upon the requirements and requests of management and the board.

The internal auditing department is an integral part of the organization and functions under the policies established by management and the board. The statement of purpose, authority, and responsibility (charter) for the internal auditing department, approved by management and accepted by the board, should be consistent with these *Standards for the Professional Practice of Internal Auditing*.

The charter should make clear the purposes of the internal auditing department, specify the unrestricted scope of its work, and declare that auditors are to have no authority or responsibility for the activities they audit.

Throughout the world internal auditing is performed in diverse environments and within organizations which vary in purpose, size, and structure. In addition, the laws and customs within various countries differ from one another. These differences may affect the practice of internal auditing in each environment. The implementation of these *Standards*, therefore, will be governed by the environment in which the internal auditing department carries out its assigned responsibilities. But compliance with the concepts enunciated by these *Standards* is essential before the responsibilities of internal auditors can be met.

"Independence," as used in these *Standards*, requires clarification. Internal auditors must be independent of the activities they audit. Such independence permits internal auditors to perform their work freely and objectively. Without independence, the desired results of internal auditing cannot be realized.

In setting these *Standards*, the following developments were considered:
1. Boards of directors are being held increasingly accountable for the adequacy and effectiveness of their organizations' systems of internal control and quality of performance.
2. Members of management are demonstrating increased acceptance of internal auditing as a means of supplying objective analyses, appraisals, recommendations, counsel, and information on the organization's controls and performance.
3. External auditors are using the results of internal audits to complement their own work where the internal auditors have provided suitable evidence of independence and adequate, professional audit work.

In the light of such developments, the purposes of these *Standards* are to:

1. Impart an understanding of the role and responsibilities of internal auditing to all levels of management, boards of directors, public bodies, external auditors, and related professional organizations
2. Establish the basis for the guidance and measurement of internal auditing performance
3. Improve the practice of internal auditing

The *Standards* differentiate among the varied responsibilities of the organization, the internal auditing department, the director of internal auditing, and internal auditors.

The five general *Standards* are expressed in italicized statements in upper case. Following each of these general *Standards* are specific standards expressed in italicized statements in lower case. Accompanying each specific standard are guidelines describing suitable means of meeting that standard. The *Standards* encompass:

1. The independence of the internal auditing department from the activities audited and the objectivity of internal auditors
2. The proficiency of internal auditors and the professional care they should exercise
3. The scope of internal auditing work
4. The performance of internal auditing assignments
5. The management of the internal auditing department

The *Standards* and the accompanying guidelines employ three terms which have been given specific meanings. These are as follows:

The term *board* includes boards of directors, audit committees of such boards, heads of agencies or legislative bodies to whom internal auditors report, boards of governors or trustees of nonprofit organizations, and any other designated governing bodies of organizations.

The terms *director of internal auditing* and *director* identify the top position in an internal auditing department.

The term *internal auditing department* includes any unit or activity within an organization which performs internal auditing functions.

SUMMARY OF GENERAL AND SPECIFIC STANDARDS FOR THE PROFESSIONAL PRACTICE OF INTERNAL AUDITING

100   **INDEPENDENCE** — *INTERNAL AUDITORS SHOULD BE INDEPENDENT OF THE ACTIVITIES THEY AUDIT.*

  110   **Organizational Status** — *The organizational status of the internal auditing department should be sufficient to permit the accomplishment of its audit responsibilities.*

  120   **Objectivity** — *Internal auditors should be objective in performing audits.*

200   **PROFESSIONAL PROFICIENCY** — *INTERNAL AUDITS SHOULD BE PERFORMED WITH PROFICIENCY AND DUE PROFESSIONAL CARE.*

  The Internal Auditing Department

  210   **Staffing** — *The internal auditing department should provide assurance that the technical proficiency and educational background of internal auditors are appropriate for the audits to be performed.*

  220   **Knowledge, Skills, and Disciplines** — *The internal auditing department should possess or should obtain the knowledge, skills, and disciplines needed to carry out its audit responsibilities.*

  230   **Supervision** — *The internal auditing department should provide assurance that internal audits are properly supervised.*

  The Internal Auditor

  240   **Compliance with Standards of Conduct** — *Internal auditors should comply with professional standards of conduct.*

  250   **Knowledge, Skills, and Disciplines** — *Internal auditors should possess the knowledge, skills, and disciplines essential to the performance of internal audits.*

  260   **Human Relations and Communications** — *Internal auditors should be skilled in dealing with people and in communicating effectively.*

  270   **Continuing Education** — *Internal auditors should maintain their technical competence through continuing education.*

  280   **Due Professional Care** — *Internal auditors should exercise due professional care in performing internal audits.*

300   **SCOPE OF WORK** — *THE SCOPE OF THE INTERNAL AUDIT SHOULD ENCOMPASS THE EXAMINATION AND EVALUATION OF THE ADEQUACY AND EFFECTIVENESS OF THE ORGANIZATION'S SYSTEM OF INTERNAL CONTROL AND THE QUALITY OF PERFORMANCE IN CARRYING OUT ASSIGNED RESPONSIBILITIES.*

  310   **Reliability and Integrity of Information** — *Internal auditors should review the reliability and integrity of financial and operating information and the means used to identify, measure, classify, and report such information.*

320 **Compliance with Policies, Plans, Procedures, Laws, and Regulations** — *Internal auditors should review the systems established to ensure compliance with those policies, plans, procedures, laws, and regulations which could have a significant impact on operations and reports and should determine whether the organization is in compliance.*

330 **Safeguarding of Assets** — *Internal auditors should review the means of safeguarding assets and, as appropriate, verify the existence of such assets.*

340 **Economical and Efficient Use of Resources** — *Internal auditors should appraise the economy and efficiency with which resources are employed.*

350 **Accomplishment of Established Objectives and Goals for Operations or Programs** — *Internal auditors should review operations or programs to ascertain whether results are consistent with established objectives and goals and whether the operations or programs are being carried out as planned.*

400 **PERFORMANCE OF AUDIT WORK** — *AUDIT WORK SHOULD INCLUDE PLANNING THE AUDIT, EXAMINING AND EVALUATING INFORMATION, COMMUNICATING RESULTS, AND FOLLOWING UP.*

410 **Planning the Audit** — *Internal auditors should plan each audit.*

420 **Examining and Evaluating Information** — *Internal auditors should collect, analyze, interpret, and document information to support audit results.*

430 **Communicating Results** — *Internal auditors should report the results of their audit work.*

440 **Following Up** — *Internal auditors should follow up to ascertain that appropriate action is taken on reported audit findings.*

500 **MANAGEMENT OF THE INTERNAL AUDITING DEPARTMENT** — *THE DIRECTOR OF INTERNAL AUDITING SHOULD PROPERLY MANAGE THE INTERNAL AUDITING DEPARTMENT.*

510 **Purpose, Authority, and Responsibility** — *The director of internal auditing should have a statement of purpose, authority, and responsibility for the internal auditing department.*

520 **Planning** — *The director of internal auditing should establish plans to carry out the responsibilities of the internal auditing department.*

530 **Policies and Procedures** — *The director of internal auditing should provide written policies and procedures to guide the audit staff.*

540 **Personnel Management and Development** — *The director of internal auditing should establish a program for selecting and developing the human resources of the internal auditing department.*

550 **External Auditors** — *The director of internal auditing should coordinate internal and external audit efforts.*

560 **Quality Assurance** — *The director of internal auditing should establish and maintain a quality assurance program to evaluate the operations of the internal auditing department.*

100   **INDEPENDENCE**

INTERNAL AUDITORS SHOULD BE INDEPENDENT
OF THE ACTIVITIES THEY AUDIT.

.01 Internal auditors are independent when they can carry out their work freely and objectively. Independence permits internal auditors to render the impartial and unbiased judgments essential to the proper conduct of audits. It is achieved through organizational status and objectivity.

110 Organizational Status

The organizational status of the internal auditing department should be sufficient to permit the accomplishment of its audit responsibilities.

.01 Internal auditors should have the support of management and of the board of directors so that they can gain the cooperation of auditees and perform their work free from interference.

.1   The director of the internal auditing department should be responsible to an individual in the organization with sufficient authority to promote independence and to ensure broad audit coverage, adequate consideration of audit reports, and appropriate action on audit recommendations.

.2   The director should have direct communication with the board. Regular communication with the board helps assure independence and provides a means for the board and the director to keep each other informed on matters of mutual interest.

.3   Independence is enhanced when the board concurs in the appointment or removal of the director of the internal auditing department.

.4   The purpose, authority, and responsibility of the internal auditing department should be defined in a formal written document (charter). The director should seek approval of the charter by management as well as acceptance by the board. The charter should (a) establish the department's position within the organization; (b) authorize access to records, personnel, and physical properties relevant to the performance of audits; and (c) define the scope of internal auditing activities.

.5   The director of internal auditing should submit annually to management for approval and to the board for its information a summary of the department's audit work schedule, staffing plan, and financial budget. The director should also submit all significant interim changes for approval and information. Audit work schedules, staffing plans, and financial budgets should inform management and the board of the scope of internal auditing work and of any limitations placed on that scope.

.6   The director of internal auditing should submit activity reports to management and to the board annually or more frequently as necessary. Activity reports should highlight significant audit findings and recommendations and should inform management and the board of any significant deviations from approved audit work schedules, staffing plans, and financial budgets, and the reasons for them.

120   Objectivity

Internal auditors should be objective in performing audits.

.01   Objectivity is an independent mental attitude which internal auditors should maintain in performing audits. Internal auditors are not to subordinate their judgment on audit matters to that of others.

.02   Objectivity requires internal auditors to perform audits in such a manner that they have an honest belief in their work product and that no significant quality compromises are made. Internal auditors are not to be placed in situations in which they feel unable to make objective professional judgments.

.1   Staff assignments should be made so that potential and actual conflicts of interest and bias are avoided. The director should periodically obtain from the audit staff information concerning potential conflicts of interest and bias.

.2   Internal auditors should report to the director any situations in which a conflict of interest or bias is present or may reasonably be inferred. The director should then reassign such auditors.

.3   Staff assignments of internal auditors should be rotated periodically whenever it is practicable to do so.

.4   Internal auditors should not assume operating responsibilities. But if on occasion management directs internal auditors to perform nonaudit work, it should be understood that they are not functioning as internal auditors. Moreover, objectivity is presumed to be impaired when internal auditors audit any activity for which they had authority or responsibility. This impairment should be considered when reporting audit results.

.5   Persons transferred to or temporarily engaged by the internal auditing department should not be assigned to audit those activities they previously performed until a reasonable period of time has elapsed. Such assignments are presumed to impair objectivity and should be considered when supervising the audit work and reporting audit results.

.6   The results of internal auditing work should be reviewed before the related audit report is released to provide reasonable assurance that the work was performed objectively.

.03   The internal auditor's objectivity is not adversely affected when the auditor recommends standards of control for systems or reviews procedures before they are implemented. Designing, installing, and operating systems are not audit functions. Also, the drafting of procedures for systems is not an audit function. Performing such activities is presumed to impair audit objectivity.

200 PROFESSIONAL PROFICIENCY

INTERNAL AUDITS SHOULD BE PERFORMED WITH
PROFICIENCY AND DUE PROFESSIONAL CARE.

.01 Professional proficiency is the responsibility of the internal auditing department and each internal auditor. The department should assign to each audit those persons who collectively possess the necessary knowledge, skills, and disciplines to conduct the audit properly.

The Internal Auditing Department
210 **Staffing**

The internal auditing department should provide assurance that the technical proficiency and educational background of internal auditors are appropriate for the audits to be performed.

.01 The director of internal auditing should establish suitable criteria of education and experience for filling internal auditing positions, giving due consideration to scope of work and level of responsibility.

.02 Reasonable assurance should be obtained as to each prospective auditor's qualifications and proficiency.

220 **Knowledge, Skills, and Disciplines**

The internal auditing department should possess or should obtain the knowledge, skills, and disciplines needed to carry out its audit responsibilities.

.01 The internal auditing staff should collectively possess the knowledge and skills essential to the practice of the profession within the organization. These attributes include proficiency in applying internal auditing standards, procedures, and techniques.

.02 The internal auditing department should have employees or use consultants who are qualified in such disciplines as accounting, economics, finance, statistics, electronic data processing, engineering, taxation, and law as needed to meet audit responsibilities. Each member of the department, however, need not be qualified in all of these disciplines.

230 **Supervision**

The internal auditing department should provide assurance that internal audits are properly supervised.

.01 The director of internal auditing is responsible for providing appropriate audit supervision. Supervision is a continuing process, beginning with planning and ending with the conclusion of the audit assignment.

.02 Supervision includes:

.1 Providing suitable instructions to subordinates at the outset of the audit and approving the audit program

.2 Seeing that the approved audit program is carried out unless deviations are both justified and authorized

.3 Determining that audit working papers adequately support the audit findings, conclusions, and reports

.4 Making sure that audit reports are accurate, objective, clear, concise, constructive, and timely

.5 Determining that audit objectives are being met

.03   Appropriate evidence of supervision should be documented and retained.

.04   The extent of supervision required will depend on the proficiency of the internal auditors and the difficulty of the audit assignment.

.05   All internal auditing assignments, whether performed by or for the internal auditing department, remain the responsibility of its director.

The Internal Auditor

240   **Compliance with Standards of Conduct**
Internal auditors should comply with professional standards of conduct.

.01   The *Code of Ethics* of The Institute of Internal Auditors sets forth standards of conduct and provides a basis for enforcement among its members. The *Code* calls for high standards of honesty, objectivity, diligence, and loyalty to which internal auditors should conform.

250   **Knowledge, Skills, and Disciplines**
Internal auditors should possess the knowledge, skills, and disciplines essential to the performance of internal audits.

.01   Each internal auditor should possess certain knowledge and skills as follows:

.1   Proficiency in applying internal auditing standards, procedures, and techniques is required in performing internal audits. Proficiency means the ability to apply knowledge to situations likely to be encountered and to deal with them without extensive recourse to technical research and assistance.

.2   Proficiency in accounting principles and techniques is required of auditors who work extensively with financial records and reports.

.3   An understanding of management principles is required to recognize and evaluate the materiality and significance of deviations from good business practice. An understanding means the ability to apply broad knowledge to situations likely to be encountered, to recognize significant deviations, and to be able to carry out the research necessary to arrive at reasonable solutions.

.4   An appreciation is required of the fundamentals of such subjects as accounting, economics, commercial law, taxation, finance, quantitative methods, and computerized information systems. An appreciation means the ability to recognize the existence of problems or potential problems and to determine the further research to be undertaken or the assistance to be obtained.

260   **Human Relations and Communications**
Internal auditors should be skilled in dealing with people and in communicating effectively.

.01   Internal auditors should understand human relations and maintain satisfactory relationships with auditees.

.02   Internal auditors should be skilled in oral and written communications so that they can clearly and effectively convey such matters

as audit objectives, evaluations, conclusions, and recommendations.

270   Continuing Education

Internal auditors should maintain their technical competence through continuing education.

.01   Internal auditors are responsible for continuing their education in order to maintain their proficiency. They should keep informed about improvements and current developments in internal auditing standards, procedures, and techniques. Continuing education may be obtained through membership and participation in professional societies; attendance at conferences, seminars, college courses, and in-house training programs; and participation in research projects.

280   Due Professional Care

Internal Auditors should exercise due professional care in performing internal audits.

.01   Due professional care calls for the application of the care and skill expected of a reasonably prudent and competent internal auditor in the same or similar circumstances. Professional care should, therefore, be appropriate to the complexities of the audit being performed. In exercising due professional care, internal auditors should be alert to the possibility of intentional wrongdoing, errors and omissions, inefficiency, waste, ineffectiveness, and conflicts of interest. They should also be alert to those conditions and activities where irregularities are most likely to occur. In addition, they should identify inadequate controls and recommend improvements to promote compliance with acceptable procedures and practices.

.02   Due care implies reasonable care and competence, not infallibility or extraordinary performance. Due care requires the auditor to conduct examinations and verifications to a reasonable extent, but does not require detailed audits of all transactions. Accordingly, the internal auditor cannot give absolute assurance that noncompliance or irregularities do not exist. Nevertheless, the possibility of material irregularities or noncompliance should be considered whenever the internal auditor undertakes an internal auditing assignment.

.03   When an internal auditor suspects wrongdoing, the appropriate authorities within the organization should be informed. The internal auditor may recommend whatever investigation is considered necessary in the circumstances. Thereafter, the auditor should follow up to see that the internal auditing department's responsibilities have been met.

.04   Exercising due professional care means using reasonable audit skill and judgment in performing the audit. To this end, the internal auditor should consider:

.1   The extent of audit work needed to achieve audit objectives

.2   The relative materiality or significance of matters to which audit procedures are applied

.3   The adequacy and effectiveness of internal controls

.4   The cost of auditing in relation to potential benefits

.05   Due professional care includes evaluating established operating standards and determining whether those standards are acceptable and are being met. When such standards are vague, authoritative interpretations should be sought. If internal auditors are required to interpret or select operating standards, they should seek agreement with auditees as to the standards needed to measure operating performance.

300 SCOPE OF WORK

*THE SCOPE OF THE INTERNAL AUDIT SHOULD ENCOMPASS
THE EXAMINATION AND EVALUATION OF THE ADEQUACY
AND EFFECTIVENESS OF THE ORGANIZATION'S SYSTEM OF
INTERNAL CONTROL AND THE QUALITY OF PERFORMANCE
IN CARRYING OUT ASSIGNED RESPONSIBILITIES.*

.01 The scope of internal auditing work, as specified in this standard, encompasses what audit work should be performed. It is recognized, however, that management and the board of directors provide general direction as to the scope of work and the activities to be audited.

.02 The purpose of the review for adequacy of the system of internal control is to ascertain whether the system established provides reasonable assurance that the organization's objectives and goals will be met efficiently and economically.

.03 The purpose of the review for effectiveness of the system of internal control is to ascertain whether the system is functioning as intended.

.04 The purpose of the review for quality of performance is to ascertain whether the organization's objectives and goals have been achieved.

.05 The primary objectives of internal control are to ensure:

.1 The reliability and integrity of information

.2 Compliance with policies, plans, procedures, laws, and regulations

.3 The safeguarding of assets

.4 The economical and efficient use of resources

.5 The accomplishment of established objectives and goals for operations or programs

310 Reliability and Integrity of Information

Internal auditors should review the reliability and integrity of financial and operating information and the means used to identify, measure, classify, and report such information.

.01 Information systems provide data for decision making, control, and compliance with external requirements. Therefore, internal auditors should examine information systems and, as appropriate, ascertain whether:

.1 Financial and operating records and reports contain accurate, reliable, timely, complete, and useful information.

.2 Controls over record keeping and reporting are adequate and effective.

320 Compliance with Policies, Plans, Procedures, Laws and Regulations

Internal auditors should review the systems established to ensure compliance with those policies, plans, procedures, laws, and regulations which could have a significant impact on operations and reports, and should determine whether the organization is in compliance.

.01 Management is responsible for establishing the systems designed to ensure compliance with such requirements as policies, plans, procedures, and applicable laws and regulations. Internal auditors are responsible for determining whether the systems are adequate and effective and whether the activities audited are complying with the appropriate requirements.

330   Safeguarding of Assets

Internal auditors should review the means of safeguarding assets and, as appropriate, verify the existence of such assets.

.01   Internal auditors should review the means used to safeguard assets from various types of losses such as those resulting from theft, fire, improper or illegal activities, and exposure to the elements.

.02   Internal auditors, when verifying the existence of assets, should use appropriate audit procedures.

340   Economical and Efficient Use of Resources

Internal auditors should appraise the economy and efficiency with which resources are employed.

.01   Management is responsible for setting operating standards to measure an activity's economical and efficient use of resources. Internal auditors are responsible for determining whether:

.1   Operating standards have been established for measuring economy and efficiency.

.2   Established operating standards are understood and are being met.

.3   Deviations from operating standards are identified, analyzed, and communicated to those responsible for corrective action.

.4   Corrective action has been taken.

.02   Audits related to the economical and efficient use of resources should identify such conditions as:

.1   Underutilized facilities

.2   Nonproductive work

.3   Procedures which are not cost justified

.4   Overstaffing or understaffing

350   Accomplishment of Established Objectives and Goals for Operations or Programs

Internal auditors should review operations or programs to ascertain whether results are consistent with established objectives and goals and whether the operations or programs are being carried out as planned.

.01   Management is responsible for establishing operating or program objectives and goals, developing and implementing control procedures, and accomplishing desired operating or program results. Internal auditors should ascertain whether such objectives and goals conform with those of the organization and whether they are being met.

.02   Internal auditors can provide assistance to managers who are developing objectives, goals, and systems by determining whether the underlying assumptions are appropriate; whether accurate, current, and relevant information is being used; and whether suitable controls have been incorporated into the operations or programs.

400   PERFORMANCE OF AUDIT WORK

AUDIT WORK SHOULD INCLUDE PLANNING THE AUDIT,
EXAMINING AND EVALUATING INFORMATION,
COMMUNICATING RESULTS, AND FOLLOWING UP.

.01   The internal auditor is responsible for planning and conducting the audit assignment, subject to supervisory review and approval.

410   Planning the Audit

Internal auditors should plan each audit.

.01   Planning should be documented and should include:

.1   Establishing audit objectives and scope of work

.2   Obtaining background information about the activities to be audited

.3   Determining the resources necessary to perform the audit

.4   Communicating with all who need to know about the audit

.5   Performing, as appropriate, an on-site survey to become familiar with the activities and controls to be audited, to identify areas for audit emphasis, and to invite auditee comments and suggestions

.6   Writing the audit program

.7   Determining how, when, and to whom audit results will be communicated

.8   Obtaining approval of the audit work plan

420   Examining and Evaluating Information

Internal auditors should collect, analyze, interpret, and document information to support audit results.

.01   The process of examining and evaluating information is as follows:

.1   Information should be collected on all matters related to the audit objectives and scope of work.

.2   Information should be sufficient, competent, relevant, and useful to provide a sound basis for audit findings and recommendations.

> *Sufficient* information is factual, adequate, and convincing so that a prudent, informed person would reach the same conclusions as the auditor.
> *Competent* information is reliable and the best attainable through the use of appropriate audit techniques.
> *Relevant* information supports audit findings and recommendations and is consistent with the objectives for the audit.
> *Useful* information helps the organization meet its goals.

.3   Audit procedures, including the testing and sampling techniques employed, should be selected in advance, where practicable, and expanded or altered if circumstances warrant.

.4   The process of collecting, analyzing, interpreting, and documenting information should be supervised to provide reasonable assurance that the auditor's objectivity is maintained and that audit goals are met.

.5 Working papers that document the audit should be prepared by the auditor and reviewed by management of the internal auditing department. These papers should record the information obtained and the analyses made and should support the bases for the findings and recommendations to be reported.

430 Communicating Results

Internal auditors should report the results of their audit work.

.1 A signed, written report should be issued after the audit examination is completed. Interim reports may be written or oral and may be transmitted formally or informally.

.2 The internal auditor should discuss conclusions and recommendations at appropriate levels of management before issuing final written reports.

.3 Reports should be objective, clear, concise, constructive, and timely.

.4 Reports should present the purpose, scope, and results of the audit; and, where appropriate, reports should contain an expression of the auditor's opinion.

.5 Reports may include recommendations for potential improvements and acknowledge satisfactory performance and corrective action.

.6 The auditee's views about audit conclusions or recommendations may be included in the audit report.

.7 The director of internal auditing or designee should review and approve the final audit report before issuance and should decide to whom the report will be distributed.

440 Following Up

Internal auditors should follow up to ascertain that appropriate action is taken on reported audit findings.

.01 Internal auditing should determine that corrective action was taken and is achieving the desired results, or that management or the board has assumed the risk of not taking corrective action on reported findings.

500   MANAGEMENT OF THE INTERNAL AUDITING DEPARTMENT

*THE DIRECTOR OF INTERNAL AUDITING SHOULD
PROPERLY MANAGE THE INTERNAL AUDITING DEPARTMENT.*

.01   The director of internal auditing is responsible for properly managing the department so that:

.1   Audit work fulfills the general purposes and responsibilities approved by management and accepted by the board.

.2   Resources of the internal auditing department are efficiently and effectively employed.

.3   Audit work conforms to the *Standards for the Professional Practice of Internal Auditing.*

510   Purpose, Authority, and Responsibility

The director of internal auditing should have a statement of purpose, authority, and responsibility for the internal auditing department.

.01   The director of internal auditing is responsible for seeking the approval of management and the acceptance by the board of a formal written document (charter) for the internal auditing department.

520   Planning

The director of internal auditing should establish plans to carry out the responsibilities of the internal auditing department.

.01   These plans should be consistent with the internal auditing department's charter and with the goals of the organization.

.02   The planning process involves establishing:

.1   Goals

.2   Audit work schedules

.3   Staffing plans and financial budgets

.4   Activity reports

.03   The *goals* of the internal auditing department should be capable of being accomplished within specified operating plans and budgets and, to the extent possible, should be measurable. They should be accompanied by measurement criteria and targeted dates of accomplishment.

.04   *Audit work schedules* should include (a) what activities are to be audited; (b) when they will be audited; and (c) the estimated time required, taking into account the scope of the audit work planned and the nature and extent of audit work performed by others. Matters to be considered in establishing audit work schedule priorities should include (a) the date and results of the last audit; (b) financial exposure; (c) potential loss and risk; (d) requests by management; (e) major changes in operations, programs, systems, and controls; (f) opportunities to achieve operating benefits; and (g) changes to and capabilities of the audit staff. The work schedules should be sufficiently flexible to cover unanticipated demands on the internal auditing department.

.05   *Staffing plans and financial budgets*, including the number of auditors and the knowledge, skills, and disciplines required to perform their work, should be determined from audit work schedules, administrative activities, education and training requirements, and audit research and development efforts.

.06   *Activity reports* should be submitted periodically to management and to the board. These reports should compare (a) performance with the department's goals and audit work schedules and (b) expenditures with financial budgets. They should explain the reasons for major variances and indicate any action taken or needed.

530   Policies and Procedures

The director of internal auditing should provide written policies and procedures to guide the audit staff.

.01   The form and content of written policies and procedures should be appropriate to the size and structure of the internal auditing department and the complexity of its work. Formal administrative and technical audit manuals may not be needed by all internal auditing departments. A small internal auditing department may be managed informally. Its audit staff may be directed and controlled through daily, close supervision and written memoranda. In a large internal auditing department, more formal and comprehensive policies and procedures are essential to guide the audit staff in the consistent compliance with the department's standards of performance.

540   Personnel Management and Development

The director of internal auditing should establish a program for selecting and developing the human resources of the internal auditing department.

.01   The program should provide for:

.1   Developing written job descriptions for each level of the audit staff

.2   Selecting qualified and competent individuals

.3   Training and providing continuing educational opportunities for each internal auditor

.4   Appraising each internal auditor's performance at least annually

.5   Providing counsel to internal auditors on their performance and professional development

550   External Auditors

The director of internal auditing should coordinate internal and external audit efforts.

.01   The internal and external audit work should be coordinated to ensure adequate audit coverage and to minimize duplicate efforts.

.02   Coordination of audit efforts involves:

.1   Periodic meetings to discuss matters of mutual interest

.2   Access to each other's audit programs and working papers

.3   Exchange of audit reports and management letters

.4   Common understanding of audit techniques, methods, and terminology

560   Quality Assurance

The director of internal auditing should establish and maintain a quality

assurance program to evaluate the operations of the internal auditing department.

.01 The purpose of this program is to provide reasonable assurance that audit work conforms with these *Standards*, the internal auditing department's charter, and other applicable standards. A quality assurance program should include the following elements:

.1 Supervision
.2 Internal reviews
.3 External reviews

.02 *Supervision* of the work of the internal auditors should be carried out continually to assure conformance with internal auditing standards, departmental policies, and audit programs.

.03 *Internal reviews* should be performed periodically by members of the internal auditing staff to appraise the quality of the audit work performed. These reviews should be performed in the same manner as any other internal audit.

.04 *External reviews* of the internal auditing department should be performed to appraise the quality of the department's operations. These reviews should be performed by qualified persons who are independent of the organization and who do not have either a real or an apparent conflict of interest. Such reviews should be conducted at least once every three years. On completion of the review, a formal, written report should be issued. The report should express an opinion as to the department's compliance with the *Standards for the Professional Practice of Internal Auditing* and, as appropriate, should include recommendations for improvement.

Statement of Responsibilities of the Internal Auditor

STATEMENT OF RESPONSIBILITIES
OF THE INTERNAL AUDITOR

NATURE

Internal Auditing is an independent appraisal activity within an organization for the review of operations as a service to management. It is a managerial control which functions by measuring and evaluating the effectiveness of other controls.

OBJECTIVE AND SCOPE

The objective of internal auditing is to assist all members of management in the effective discharge of their responsibilities, by furnishing them with analyses, appraisals, recommendations and pertinent comments concerning the activities reviewed. The internal auditor is concerned with any phase of business activity where he can be of service to management. This involves going beyond the accounting and financial records to obtain a full understanding of the operations under review. The attainment of this overall objective involves such activities as:

— Reviewing and appraising the soundness, adequacy, and application of accounting, financial, and other operating controls, and promoting effective control at reasonable cost.
— Ascertaining the extent of compliance with established policies, plans, and procedures.
— Ascertaining the extent to which company assets are accounted for and safeguarded from losses of all kinds.
— Ascertaining the reliability of management data developed within the organization.
— Appraising the quality of performance in carrying out assigned responsibilities.
— Recommending operating improvements.

RESPONSIBILITY AND AUTHORITY

The responsibilities of internal auditing in the organization should be clearly established by management policy. The related authority should provide the internal auditor full access to all of the organization's records, properties, and personnel relevant to the subject under review. The internal auditor should be free to review and appraise policies, plans, procedures, and records.

The internal auditor's responsibilities should be:

— To inform and advise management, and to discharge this responsibility in a manner that is consistent with the Code of Ethics of The Institute of Internal Auditors.
— To coordinate his activities with others so as to best achieve his audit objectives and the objectives of the organization.

In performing his functions, an internal auditor has no direct responsibility for nor authority over any of the activities which he reviews. Therefore, the internal audit review and appraisal does not in any way relieve other persons in the organization of the responsibilities assigned to them.

INDEPENDENCE

Independence is essential to the effectiveness of internal auditing. This independence is obtained primarily through organizational status and objectivity:

- The organizational status of the internal auditing function and the support accorded to it by management are major determinants of its range and value. The head of the internal auditing function, therefore, should be responsible to an officer whose authority is sufficient to assure both a broad range of audit coverage and the adequate consideration of and effective action on the audit findings and recommendations.

- Objectivity is essential to the audit function. Therefore, an internal auditor should not develop and install procedures, prepare records, or engage in any other activity which he would normally review and appraise and which could reasonably be construed to compromise his independence. His objectivity need not be adversely affected, however, by his determination and recommendation of the standards of control to be applied in the development of systems and procedures under his review.

The Statement of Responsibilities of the Internal Auditor was originally issued by The Institute of Internal Auditors in 1947. The continuing development of the profession has resulted in two revisions, in 1957 and 1971. The current statement embodies the concepts previously established and includes such changes as are deemed advisable in light of the present status of the profession.

Appendix C

Code of Ethics

THE INSTITUTE OF INTERNAL AUDITORS, INC.

Code of Ethics

INTRODUCTION:

Recognizing that ethics are an important consideration in the practice of internal auditing and that the moral principles followed by members of THE INSTITUTE OF INTERNAL AUDITORS, INC. should be formalized, the Board of Directors at its regular meeting in New Orleans on December 13, 1968, received and adopted the following resolution:

WHEREAS, the members of THE INSTITUTE OF INTERNAL AUDITORS, INC. represent the profession of internal auditing; and

WHEREAS, managements rely on the profession of internal auditing to assist in the fulfillment of their management stewardship; and

WHEREAS, said members must maintain high standards of conduct, honor and character in order to carry on proper and meaningful internal auditing practice;

THEREFORE BE IT RESOLVED that a Code of Ethics be now set forth outlining the standards of professional behavior for the guidance of each member of THE INSTITUTE OF INTERNAL AUDITORS, INC.

In accordance with this resolution, the Board of Directors further approved of the principles set forth.

INTERPRETATION OF PRINCIPLES:

The provisions of this Code of Ethics cover basic principles in the various disciplines of internal auditing practice. A member shall realize that individual judgment is required in the application of these principles. He has a responsibility to conduct himself so that his good faith and integrity should not be open to question. While having due regard for the limit of his technical skills, he will promote the highest possible internal auditing standards to the end of advancing the interest of his company or organization.

ARTICLES:

I. A member shall have an obligation to exercise honesty, objectivity and diligence in the performance of his duties and responsibilities.

II. A member, in holding the trust of his employer, shall exhibit loyalty in all matters pertaining to the affairs of the employer or to whomever he may be rendering a service. However, a member shall not knowingly be a party to any illegal or improper activity.

III. A member shall refrain from entering into any activity which may be in conflict with the interest of his employer or which would prejudice his ability to carry out objectively his duties and responsibilities.

IV. A member shall not accept a fee or a gift from an employee, a client, a customer or a business associate of his employer without the knowledge and consent of his senior management.

V. A member shall be prudent in the use of information acquired in the course of his duties. He shall not use confidential information for any personal gain or in a manner which would be detrimental to the welfare of his employer.

VI. A member, in expressing an opinion, shall use all reasonable care to obtain sufficient factual evidence to warrant such expression. In his reporting, a member shall reveal such material facts known to him which, if not revealed, could either distort the report of the results of operations under review or conceal unlawful practice.

VII. A member shall continually strive for improvement in the proficiency and effectiveness of his service.

VIII. A member shall abide by the Bylaws and uphold the objectives of THE INSTITUTE OF INTERNAL AUDITORS, INC. In the practice of his profession, he shall be ever mindful of his obligation to maintain the high standard of competence, morality and dignity which THE INSTITUTE OF INTERNAL AUDITORS, INC. and its members have established.

The Common Body of Knowledge for Internal Auditors

Enormous challenges for many trained traditional disciplines have emerged in the past decade. Professional organizations and their members are giving careful thought to their roles in the future. The established professions of medicine, public accounting and law are making greater efforts in research, education, and the performance of their professional services. At the same time, groups offering all types of specialized services are accelerating the pace to obtain professional recognition and status.

Since its formal organization in 1941, The Institute of Internal Auditors has come a long way. The profession has successfully reacted to change and is performing valuable services for management. The initiative and leadership of our profession is reflected in our research, our publications and our technical conferences. The formation of a Professional Development Committee in 1966 reflected the need to study the merits of a certification program.

The establishment of the Cadmus Education Foundation was also a significant milestone in the educational activities of The Institute. All of the accomplishments to date have strived to achieve the objective of the Institute: "To promote the recognition and the practice of internal auditing throughout the world."

One of the important characteristics of a profession is a common body of knowledge. A body of knowledge forms the conceptual foundation of a profession and serves as a basis for education, training, recruiting and testing the competence of those who wish to enter a professional field. It also provides a framework for dialogue between the profession and those it serves.

In 1971, a subcommittee of the International Education Committee was formed to "coordinate with the Professional Development Committee and the Research Committee in studying basic curricula and areas for examination under the certification program."

The first task undertaken by the subcommittee was to research the body of knowledge of the internal auditing profession and to identify the areas of common knowledge of internal auditors. A review was made of relevant literature from a wide spectrum of articles and professional magazines including *The Internal Auditor*. This literature represented many professional bodies in the business world. They ranged from the public accounting bodies in the United States, Canada, the United Kingdom, Australia and New Zealand to the management accounting societies as well as other organizations such as the Association for Systems Management, Data Processing Management Association, Administrative Management Society, Chartered Institute of Secretaries (U.K. and Canada), American Society for Production and Inventory Control, etc.

In addition, a detailed review was made of the common body of knowledge and educational guidelines of a number of professional organizations in the management field. These included the following certified or accredited professions:

- American Institute of Certified Public Accountants (C.P.A.)

- Canadian Institute of Chartered Accountants (C.A.)
- Canadian Association of Management Consultants (M.I.M.C.)
- Society of Industrial Accountants in Canada (R.I.A.)
- Joint Diploma in Management Accounting Services of the British Accounting Societies (J. Dip. M.A.)
- Certificate in Management Information of the Institute of Chartered Accountants in England and Wales and the Institute of Chartered Accountants in Ireland

A review was also made of the common body of knowledge and education guidelines of the following noncertified or nonaccredited professions:

- Association of Consulting Management Engineers (U.S.)
- National Association of Accountants (This body has since organized an Institute of Management and a certification program in the U.S.)
- Federal Government Accountants Association (U.S.)

A questionnaire was developed to identify the common body of knowledge for internal auditors. This questionnaire was distributed to The Institute of Internal Auditors' international officers and directors and to the chairmen and committee members of all international committees, representing 100 members of the organization. Seventy-five percent of the questionnaires were completed and tabulated.

The survey revealed the following broad areas of the *Common Body of Knowledge for Internal Auditors*:

1. Accounting and Finance
2. Auditing
3. Behavioral Sciences
4. Communications
5. Computer Systems and Equipment
6. Economics
7. Legal Aspects of Business
8. The Management Process and Management Activities
9. Quantitative Methods
10. Systems and Procedures

ACCOUNTING AND FINANCE

Accounting is generally referred to as the "language of business." An effective accounting system is the major quantitative information and control system in most organizations. It provides information for three broad purposes:

- Internal reporting to management for use in planning and controlling current operations.
- Internal reporting to management for use in formulating overall policies and long-range plans and in making special decisions.
- External reporting to stockholders, governments and other outside parties.

In the past, internal auditing was closely allied with the public accounting profession and placed a major emphasis on financial audits and the attest function. The attest function lends credibility to the representations of one party to another. It is generally used for external reporting in all business organizations but seldom used for internal reporting in large public companies.

Management accounting places its emphasis on internal reporting. It is the accounting for planning and control. The management-oriented internal audit emphasizes that internal auditing and external auditing are distinct fields and require different emphasis on financial and managerial accounting.

The modern internal auditor recognizes that his function is not to attest to management but rather to assure them on the reliability of internal reporting. His service is to all management in the organization.

The *Common Body of Knowledge for Internal Auditors* includes the fundamental concepts of accounting and finance with a good working knowledge of:

- **Financial Accounting**
  Development of accounting theory, valuation and measurement of income, financial statement presentation, government and other regulations and professional accounting body recommendations (AICPA/CICA), current issues and developments, current assets and liabilities, working capital and flow of funds, long-lived assets, shareholders equity.
- **Managerial Accounting**
  Elements of costs, job order and process cost systems, budgeting, standard costs and analysis of variances, cost/volume/profit relationships, variable costing, relevant costs, cost analysis applied to decision making, capital budgeting, current developments in management accounting.
- **Finance**
  Planning concepts and techniques, control concepts and techniques, capital investment analysis, performance measurement.

AUDITING

Auditing can be defined as the examination of information by a third party other than the preparer or user with the intent of establishing its reliability. As applied to internal auditing, it extends beyond the examination of information to the review of all business operations so as to ascertain the soundness, adequacy and application of management controls and appraising the quality of performance with the organization. The modern internal auditor monitors the complete network of management controls by subjecting all operations to an objective examination.

The Common Body of Knowledge for Internal Auditors must be substantively oriented toward management-oriented auditing as opposed to the traditional external-audit type.

The internal auditor must have a good working knowledge of:

- **Auditing Theory**
  Nature and purpose of auditing; responsibilities of the internal auditor; relationship between external and internal auditing; internal control; fraud; procedures for the audit of balance sheets items, particularly cash, accounts receivable, inventories; internal auditing standards; code of ethics; internal audit reports.
- **Audit Tools and Techniques**
  Fraud investigations; flowcharting and statistical sampling; audits of business operations; manufacturing, inventory, procurement, sales and advertising, information systems, planning and control procedures, and managerial performance; current developments in internal auditing.
- **Audit Administration**
  Administration of the Audit Department; organizing, planning and controlling; staff selection, development and evaluation; coordination with outside auditors; selling internal auditing to management; administration of the audit assignment; planning the audit, conducting the audit, reviewing the progress of the audit, reporting the results of the audit.

BEHAVIORAL SCIENCES AND COMMUNICATIONS

There is a growing body of theory and practice about individual and group behavior, organizational structure, and the process of individual and organizational decision making. In appraising performance, the internal auditor must understand individual and group behavior, the decision process, and organization theory.

Effective communication is an indispensable skill, particularly for a professional. The internal auditor must be proficient in analyzing, appraising, recommending and making pertinent comments about the operations under review. He must be able to express himself in a clear, constructive, coherent and comprehensive manner.

The common body of knowledge required of internal auditors commends a good working knowledge of:

- **Behavioral Sciences**
  Conceptual foundation of organizational behavior, the individual in the organization, the group in the organization, structural aspects of organizational behavior, society as a social system, social psychology, and the prediction of human behavior
- **Communications**
  Effective communication: putting ideas together, using communications media, audiovisual media, written media, human media.

COMPUTERS AND SYSTEMS

With the advent of the computer, management has a complex tool of vast potential. The modern internal auditor cannot escape involvement with the computer. It is becoming one of the principal analytical tools and is involved in every phase of management activity. The *Common Body of Knowledge for Internal Auditors* includes a good working knowledge of the capabilities and limitations of computers and an awareness and understanding of the control procedures required. It also includes sound knowledge of the audit techniques applicable to the computer environment.

- **Computers**
  Fundamental concepts of using a computer; the components of a computer system; computer programming and remote terminals; business information processing; current developments in computer technology.
- **Computer Audit**
  EDP controls; auditing in the EDP environment; special audit problems; feasibility studies and systems conversion; introduction to systems design and analysis; current developments in auditing EDP systems.

ECONOMICS

Economic forces which affect every organization are measured and communicated through accounting. As a managerial control, the internal auditor must understand the economic forces that affect the organization, the relationship of price to demand, the behavior of costs, the cost concepts, productivity, and the role of government in the regulation of business. The common body of knowledge includes:

- **Economics**
  The basic forces at work in the economic system; the concepts of national output and income; aggregate employment and the general level of prices;

the role of money and the banking system; fiscal and monetary policies; international economics; economic growth and development.

- **Economic Analysis of Business**
  The economic theory of the firm and its application to managerial analysis and decision making. This includes market theory, production theory, pricing, costs, demand analysis, and market forecasting for operations planning.

THE LEGAL ASPECTS OF BUSINESS

A conceptual knowledge of law is inseparable from the knowledge of other subjects related to the business environment. There are legal implications with customers, suppliers, employees, and the public at large. There are legal problems related to taxation, unions, investments, franchises, patents, organizations, etc.

The common body of knowledge required by the internal auditor should be sufficiently broad so that he can recognize, at the least, that a problem has legal aspects. He should be able to apply the underlying principles to auditing situations and to seek legal counsel or recommend it be sought whenever appropriate.

MANAGEMENT AND MANAGEMENT ACTIVITIES

The 1971 *Statement of Responsibilities of the Internal Auditor* clearly states: "The internal auditor is concerned with any phase of business activity where he can be of service to management." As a "managerial control which functions by measuring and evaluating the effectiveness of other controls," the internal auditor must know and understand management and the activities of management.

The internal auditor must have sound knowledge of the conceptual framework of management and the management process—planning, organizing, staffing, directing, and controlling. He must be very knowledgeable about professional management—present and future.

But that is not enough! The internal auditor must also have good knowledge of the specialized activities of management. A specialized activity area can be defined as a group of management functions which, because of common objectives, common skill requirements, or merely management choice, are usually directed by a member of top management with specialized knowledge and skills in the area. The management activities are generally understood to include external relations, finance and control, marketing, personnel administration, production, secretarial and legal, and research and development.

Each specialized management activity has a number of functions and subfunctions. For example, the production activity could involve the functions of plant engineering, industrial engineering, purchasing, production planning and control, manufacturing, and quality control. The purchasing function could then be broken down into subfunctions such as buying, expediting, purchase records and files, purchase research, and salvage sales.

The internal auditor does not require the full depth of knowledge of the specialist in a particular activity or function. He is concerned with the elements of control; e.g., the organization, the systems of authorization and recording, the sound practices to be followed in the performance of duties and functions and a quality of personnel commensurate with responsibilities.

The *Common Body of Knowledge for Internal Auditors* includes a sound knowledge of the management process and of the specialized activity areas of business. The knowledge and ability to recognize the relative importance and proper or logical location of each function and subfunction is essential, particularly in respect to the means of control available to management in each function.

QUANTITATIVE METHODS

The expanding use of quantitative sciences and the knowledge "explosion" of tools and techniques for decision making, forecasting, formal planning, and performance evaluation requires knowledge of mathematics, statistics, and probability. The expanding use of the computer in its application to business problems is continually forcing the expansion of knowledge in the quantitative sciences.

The *Common Body of Knowledge for Internal Auditors* is conceptual rather than manipulative. It includes an appreciation of the mathematical techniques and their application to business situations and problems.

- **Business Mathematics**
  Algebra; organizing statistical data; charting and graphs; simple and compound interest. Bonds, amortization and sinking funds; investment decision making. Annuities, perpetuities, matrices, and the algebra of sets.
- **Information Systems: Analysis, Design and Implementation**
  Information theory; systems concepts; data processing systems. Information technology; planning analysis and implementation. Post-installation evaluation and systems audit.

SYSTEMS AND PROCEDURES

The field of systems and procedures is an integral part of the knowledge of any management-oriented person. Every person who supervises, directs, or administers the activities of subordinates has an inherent responsibility for the systems that he and his subordinates employ. Management control operates through systems and procedures.

The internal auditor must have a good working knowledge of systems and procedures in order to review and appraise the soundness, adequacy, and applications of controls and to promote effective control at reasonable cost. The body of knowledge includes the systems environment; gathering and analyzing the facts; work simplification; work measurement; work sampling; office and plant layout; forms control and records management; and office mechanization.

LEVELS OF KNOWLEDGE

The results of the questionnaire developed by the subcommittee are tabled in Exhibit I. For purposes of identifying the levels of knowledge required, the definitions used were:

Level One

- Appreciation of the broad nature and the fundamentals involved.
- Ability to recognize the existence of the likelihood of existence of special features and problems in various business transactions and to determine what further study or research must be undertaken under various conditions.

Level Two

- Sound appreciation of the broad aspects of practices and procedures and awareness of the problems relating to more detailed aspects thereof.
- The ability to apply such broad knowledge to situations likely to be encountered, to recognize the more detailed aspects which must be considered and to carry out research and studies necessary to come to a reasonable solution.

Level Three

- Sound understanding of principles, practices and procedures.
- The ability to apply such knowledge to situations likely to be encountered and to deal with all aspects thereof without extensive recourse to technical research and assistance.

The results of the questionnaire identified the broad areas of the common body of knowledge. If internal auditors run true to form, many will question the levels of knowledge indicated by the questionnaire results. For example, the levels of

Exhibit 1   Results of Questionnaire Regarding Common Body of Knowledge for Internal Auditors

	Weighted Average	Level One	Level Two	Level Three
1.00 ACCOUNTING AND FINANCE	2.18			
1.01 Elementary Accounting	2.64			
1.02 Financial Accounting	2.23			
1.03 Cost Accounting	1.89			
1.04 Accounting for Management Planning and Control	1.97			
2.00 AUDITING	2.31			
2.01 Nature of Internal Auditing	2.47			
2.02 Administration of Internal Audit Dept.	1.95			
2.03 Administration of Internal Audit Assignment	2.30			
2.04 Internal Control	2.72			
2.05 The Auditor and His Environment	2.01			
2.06 Tools and Techniques of Internal Audit	2.39			
3.00 BEHAVIORAL SCIENCES	1.43			
4.00 COMMUNICATIONS	1.97			
5.00 COMPUTERS AND SYSTEMS	1.81			
5.01 Computer Concepts	1.68			
5.02 Computer Controls	1.91			
5.03 Systems Development Controls	1.69			
5.04 Organization Controls	1.84			
5.05 Procedural Controls	1.80			
5.06 Audit Techniques	1.91			
6.00 ECONOMICS	0.89			
6.01 Elementary Macro-Economics	0.89			
6.02 Elementary Micro-Economics	0.95			
6.03 The Monetary System	0.84			
7.00 LEGAL ASPECTS OF BUSINESS	1.27			
7.01 Commercial Law	1.35			
7.02 Taxation	1.19			
8.00 MANAGEMENT AND THE MANAGEMENT FUNCTIONS	1.38			
8.01 Conceptual Framework of Management	1.51			
8.02 Management Process of Planning	1.42			
8.03 Management Process of Organizing	1.45			
8.04 Management Process of Staffing	1.27			
8.05 Management Process of Directing	1.36			
8.06 Management Process of Controlling	1.64			
8.07 Managers and the Changing Environment	1.00			

	Weighted Average	Level One	Level Two	Level Three
8.08 EXTERNAL RELATIONS	0.81			
8.081 Communications and Information	1.00			
8.082 Public Activities Coordination	0.62			
8.09 FINANCE AND CONTROL	1.74			
8.091 Finance	1.54			
8.092 Control	1.93			
8.10 MARKETING	0.91			
8.101 Marketing Research	0.91			
8.102 Advertising	0.76			
8.103 Sales Promotion	0.72			
8.104 Sales Planning	0.84			
8.105 Physical Distribution	1.31			
8.11 PERSONNEL ADMINISTRATION	0.93			
8.111 Employment	0.89			
8.112 Wage and Salary Administration	0.95			
8.113 Industrial Relations	0.88			
8.114 Organizational Planning & Development	1.04			
8.115 Employee Services	0.88			
8.12 PRODUCTION	1.11			
8.121 Plant Engineering	0.85			
8.122 Industrial Engineering	1.07			
8.123 Purchasing	1.45			
8.124 Production Planning and Control	1.30			
8.125 Manufacturing	0.89			
8.126 Quality Control	1.14			
8.13 SECRETARIAL AND LEGAL	0.92			
8.131 Secretarial	0.91			
8.132 Legal	0.91			
8.14 RESEARCH AND DEVELOPMENT	0.67			
8.141 Research	0.71			
8.142 Development	0.66			
8.143 Product Engineering	0.64			
9.00 QUANTITATIVE METHODS	1.21			
9.01 Analyses	1.08			
9.02 Decision-Making	1.30			
9.03 Advanced Information Systems	1.24			
10.00 SYSTEMS AND PROCEDURES	1.61			

knowledge for computers and systems or for quantitative methods may be judged too low by the well-educated, new generation of practitioners.

The subcommittee was also concerned about some of the results obtained in various areas. Our judgment is that the results may reflect more accurately the present level of knowledge existing in the profession than what that level should be. It may be more accurate to say that it reflects the fact that the large majority of the respondents were educated in the pre-sputnik era. However, we suggest that it does show the present standards of the profession. The standards that should apply tomorrow and in the future will undoubtedly be different in some respects.

The draft of the common body of knowledge as presented by the subcommittee was discussed at the joint meeting, June 17, 1972, of the International Education Committee with the Professional Development and the Research committees. Members present unanimously agreed that the committees involved "accept and support the Common Body of Knowledge study as an initial step in developing educational requirements for internal auditors." It was also agreed that the study should serve as a basis for The Institute's certification program. (Subsequent to the meeting, the Board of Directors approved a certification program for Institute members.)

The Institute of Internal Auditors has taken one more important step on the road to achieving professional identity.

There may be a few skeptics in our profession who say that there cannot be a common body of knowledge. Because of the many disparate views held by managements from industry to industry, or even from one company to another in the same industry, and, also, because some internal auditors keep saying, for example, that an auditor in the banking business cannot possibly require the same basic knowledge as the auditor in a manufacturing industry, differences of opinion will remain. To these skeptics in management and in the profession, let us recall the recent words of William L. Campfield in *The Internal Auditor*: "Every professional group has at some time or other been faced with a 'crossroads type' question, namely: 'Should we continue to move ahead aggressively and run the risk of being accused of moving too fast and too far into areas in which we may not be fully competent, or should we travel the road of caution and consolidation of our prior gains?' Although a middle road can always be found or, if necessary, constructed for any problematical situation, I would opt for pushing ahead aggressively. Remember the ancient adage: 'The beaches of time are covered with the bleached bones of those who having rested at the shores there perished.' "

Index

About the Author

Mr. Seth Allcorn has been the Administrative Manager for the Department of Medicine, University of Missouri, Columbia Medical School for 4 years. Prior to this appointment he was, for 3 years, an internal auditor for the University of Missouri. Mr. Allcorn has published articles on internal auditing in hospitals.